POST-VIETNAM DIOXIN EXPOSURE IN AGENT ORANGE–CONTAMINATED C-123 AIRCRAFT

Committee to Evaluate the Potential Exposure to
Agent Orange/TCDD Residue and
Level of Risk of Adverse Health Effects for
Aircrew of Post-Vietnam C-123 Aircraft

Board on the Health of Select Populations

INSTITUTE OF MEDICINE
OF THE NATIONAL ACADEMIES

THE NATIONAL ACADEMIES PRESS
Washington, D.C.
www.nap.edu

THE NATIONAL ACADEMIES PRESS 500 Fifth Street, NW Washington, DC 20001

NOTICE: The project that is the subject of this report was approved by the Governing Board of the National Research Council, whose members are drawn from the councils of the National Academy of Sciences, the National Academy of Engineering, and the Institute of Medicine. The members of the committee responsible for the report were chosen for their special competences and with regard for appropriate balance.

This study was supported by Contract/Grant No. VA241-P-2024 between the National Academy of Sciences and the Department of Veterans Affairs. Any opinions, findings, conclusions, or recommendations expressed in this publication are those of the author(s) and do not necessarily reflect the views of the organizations or agencies that provided support for the project.

International Standard Book Number-13: 978-0-309-30890-8
International Standard Book Number-10: 0-309-30890-9

Additional copies of this report are available for sale from the National Academies Press, 500 Fifth Street, NW, Keck 360, Washington, DC 20001; (800) 624-6242 or (202) 334-3313; http://www.nap.edu.

For more information about the Institute of Medicine, visit the IOM home page at: **www.iom.edu.**

Printed in the United States of America

The serpent has been a symbol of long life, healing, and knowledge among almost all cultures and religions since the beginning of recorded history. The serpent adopted as a logotype by the Institute of Medicine is a relief carving from ancient Greece, now held by the Staatliche Museen in Berlin.

Suggested citation: IOM (Institute of Medicine). 2015. *Post-Vietnam Dioxin Exposure in Agent Orange–Contaminated C-123 Aircraft.* Washington, DC: The National Academies Press.

"Knowing is not enough; we must apply.
Willing is not enough; we must do."
—Goethe

INSTITUTE OF MEDICINE
OF THE NATIONAL ACADEMIES

Advising the Nation. Improving Health.

THE NATIONAL ACADEMIES

Advisers to the Nation on Science, Engineering, and Medicine

The **National Academy of Sciences** is a private, nonprofit, self-perpetuating society of distinguished scholars engaged in scientific and engineering research, dedicated to the furtherance of science and technology and to their use for the general welfare. Upon the authority of the charter granted to it by the Congress in 1863, the Academy has a mandate that requires it to advise the federal government on scientific and technical matters. Dr. Ralph J. Cicerone is president of the National Academy of Sciences.

The **National Academy of Engineering** was established in 1964, under the charter of the National Academy of Sciences, as a parallel organization of outstanding engineers. It is autonomous in its administration and in the selection of its members, sharing with the National Academy of Sciences the responsibility for advising the federal government. The National Academy of Engineering also sponsors engineering programs aimed at meeting national needs, encourages education and research, and recognizes the superior achievements of engineers. Dr. C. D. Mote, Jr. is president of the National Academy of Engineering.

The **Institute of Medicine** was established in 1970 by the National Academy of Sciences to secure the services of eminent members of appropriate professions in the examination of policy matters pertaining to the health of the public. The Institute acts under the responsibility given to the National Academy of Sciences by its congressional charter to be an adviser to the federal government and, upon its own initiative, to identify issues of medical care, research, and education. Dr. Victor J. Dzau is president of the Institute of Medicine.

The **National Research Council** was organized by the National Academy of Sciences in 1916 to associate the broad community of science and technology with the Academy's purposes of furthering knowledge and advising the federal government. Functioning in accordance with general policies determined by the Academy, the Council has become the principal operating agency of both the National Academy of Sciences and the National Academy of Engineering in providing services to the government, the public, and the scientific and engineering communities. The Council is administered jointly by both Academies and the Institute of Medicine. Dr. Ralph J. Cicerone and Dr. C. D. Mote, Jr., are chair and vice chair, respectively, of the National Research Council.

www.national-academies.org

COMMITTEE TO EVALUATE THE POTENTIAL EXPOSURE TO AGENT ORANGE/TCDD RESIDUE AND LEVEL OF RISK OF ADVERSE HEALTH EFFECTS FOR AIRCREW OF POST-VIETNAM C-123 AIRCRAFT

ROBERT F. HERRICK (*Chair*), Harvard School of Public Health
ROBERT CANALES, University of Arizona
KENNY S. CRUMP, Independent Consultant
MELISSA GONZALES, University of New Mexico
JOHN C. KISSEL, University of Washington
LINDA A. McCAULEY, Emory University
CLIFFORD P. WEISEL, Rutgers University

IOM Staff

MARY BURR PAXTON, Co-study Director, Senior Program Officer
JENNIFER A. COHEN, Co-study Director, Program Officer
HEATHER L. CHIARELLO, Research Associate
FREDERICK J. ERDTMANN, Director, Board on the Health of Select Populations

Reviewers

This report has been reviewed in draft form by individuals chosen for their diverse perspectives and technical expertise, in accordance with procedures approved by the National Research Council's Report Review Committee. The purpose of this independent review is to provide candid and critical comments that will assist the institution in making its published report as sound as possible and to ensure that the report meets institutional standards for objectivity, evidence, and responsiveness to the study charge. The review comments and draft manuscript remain confidential to protect the integrity of the deliberative process. We wish to thank the following individuals for their review of this report:

Richard A. Fenske, University of Washington
Michael A. Gallo, University of Medicine and Dentistry of New Jersey–Robert Wood Johnson Medical School
Melissa J. Perry, George Washington University
Martin A. Philbert, University of Michigan
Dale Sandler, National Institute of Environmental Health Sciences
Lauren Zeise, California Environmental Protection Agency

Although the reviewers listed above have provided many constructive comments and suggestions, they were not asked to endorse the conclusions or recommendations nor did they see the final draft of the report before its release. The review of this report was overseen by **Kristine M. Gebbie,** Flinders University of South Australia. Appointed by the National Research and the

Institute of Medicine, she was responsible for making certain that an independent examination of this report was carried out in accordance with institutional procedures and that all review comments were carefully considered. Responsibility for the final content of this report rests entirely with the authoring committee and the institution.

Acknowledgments

This report was greatly enhanced by the participants of the workshop that was held as part of this study. The committee would like to acknowledge the efforts of those who gave presentations and who provided materials to the committee during the course of the study's information-gathering period: Wesley Carter (C-123 Veterans Association), Jeffrey Driver (RiskScience.net), Patrick Finley (Sandia National Laboratories), Harry Heist II (Air Mobility Command Museum, Dover, Delaware), Peter Kahn (AESOP, Rutgers University), Peter Lurker (Germantown Consultants, LLC), Thomas McKone (University of California, Berkeley), William Nazaroff (University of California, Berkeley), Brian Nicklas (National Air and Space Museum Archives), Thomas Sinks (Agency for Toxic Substances and Disease Registry), Jeanne Stellman (Columbia University), and Alvin Young (A.L. Young Consulting, Inc.). The information that was provided helped to set the stage for fruitful discussions in the closed session that followed. The committee greatly appreciates the contribution of Roberta Wedge (Institute of Medicine) in providing experienced, but fresh eyes to the report. The committee would also like to acknowledge and thank Chensheng (Alex) Lu (Harvard School of Public Health) for his participation as a committee member before resigning in September 2014.

Contents

Acronyms and Abbreviations xiii

Summary 1

1 Introduction 11

2 TCDD: Physicochemical Properties and Health Guidelines 16

3 Air Force Use of the C-123 Provider: Background and Sampling Data 27

4 Evaluation of Assessments of Possible Exposure of Air Force Reservists from Service in Operation Ranch Hand C-123s 47

5 Summary of Findings 72

References 79

Appendixes

A Public Agendas from Committee Meetings 87

B History and Sampling of C-123s in the United States After Spraying Herbicides in Vietnam 91

C Committee Biographies 100

Acronyms and Abbreviations

2,4-D	2,4-dichlorophenoxyacetic acid
2,4,5-T	2,4,5-trichlorophenoxyacetic acid
ADI	acceptable daily intake
AF (USAF)	US Air Force
AFB	Air Force Base
AFHS	Air Force Health Study
AHR	aryl hydrocarbon receptor
AMARC	Aerospace Maintenance and Regeneration Center
AMARG	Aerospace Maintenance and Regeneration Group
AME	aero-medical evacuation
AO	Agent Orange (general term for all herbicide formulations containing TCDD)
atm	atmosphere (measure for vapor pressure)
ATSDR	Agency for Toxic Substances and Disease Registry
CAG	Cancer Assessment Group (EPA)
CHPPM	US Army Center for Health Promotion and Preventive Medicine
CVA	C-123 Veterans Association
ECG	electrocardiogram
EPA	US Environmental Protection Agency
HO	Herbicide Orange (equivalent to Agent Orange)

IOM	Institute of Medicine
LOAEL	lowest-observed-adverse-effect level
lpm	liters per minute
MAP	Military Assistance Program
MASDC	Military Aircraft Storage and Disposal Center
MDI	mean daily intake
mg/m^3	milligrams per cubic meter
NAS	National Academy of Sciences
ng/m^2	nanograms per square meter
NIEHS	National Institute of Environmental Health Sciences
NIOSH	National Institute for Occupational Safety and Health
NMDOH	New Mexico Department of Health
NOEL	no-observed-effect level
NRC	National Research Council
ORH	Operation Ranch Hand (military codename for operation that sprayed herbicides during the Vietnam War)
ORH C-123	UC-123 aircraft formerly used in ORH
PCB	polychlorinated biphenyl
PCDD	polychlorinated dibenzo-*p*-dioxin
PCDF	polychlorinated dibenzofuran
ppm	parts per million
PUF	polyurethane foam (vapor phase collection method)
QA/QC	quality assurance/quality control
RfD	noncancer reference dose
RH	Ranch Hand (name for individuals who served in ORH)
SVOC	semi-volatile organic compound
SWSL	surface wipe screening level
TAG	Tactical Airlift Group
TAS	Tactical Airlift Squadron
TC	transfer coefficient
TCDD	2,3,7,8-tetrachlorodibenzo-*p*-dioxin
TDI	tolerable daily intake
TEF	Toxicity Equivalency Factor
TEQ	Toxicity Equivalency Quotient (weighted total of TEFs)
TG 312	Technical Guide 312 (CHPPM, 2009)

TSCA	Toxic Substances Control Act
μg/kg	microgram per kilogram
μg/kg-d	microgram per kilogram per day (format for "mass per kilogram-body weight per time unit")
μg/m^2	microgram per square meter (= 0.01 μg/100 cm^2)
USAF	US Air Force
USAFSAM	US Air Force School of Aerospace Medicine
VA	Department of Veterans Affairs
VAO	Veterans and Agent Orange (IOM report series)
WHO	World Health Organization
WTC	World Trade Center
y_0	gas-phase concentration immediately above contaminated surface

Summary

BACKGROUND

From 1972 to 1982, approximately 1,500–2,100 US Air Force (AF) Reserve personnel trained and worked on C-123 aircraft that had formerly been used to spray herbicides in Vietnam as part of Operation Ranch Hand (ORH). After becoming aware that some of the aircraft on which they had worked had previously served this purpose, some of these AF Reservists applied to the US Department of Veterans Affairs (VA) for compensatory coverage under the Agent Orange (AO) Act of 1991. The AO Act provides health care and disability coverage for health conditions that have been deemed presumptively service-related for herbicide exposure during the Vietnam War. The VA denied the applications on the basis that these veterans were ineligible because as non-Vietnam-era veterans or as Vietnam-era veterans without "boots on the ground" service in Vietnam, they were not covered by the AO Act. However, with the knowledge that some air and wipe samples taken between 1979 and 2009 from some of the C-123s used in ORH showed the presence of AO residues, representatives of the C-123 Veterans Association began a concerted effort to reverse VA's position and obtain coverage.

In early 2014, the VA contracted with the Institute of Medicine (IOM) to evaluate whether or not service in these ORH C-123s could have plausibly resulted in exposures detrimental to the health of these AF Reservists. The IOM was asked to assemble an expert committee to address this question qualitatively, but in a scientific and evidence-based fashion. The resulting committee was explicitly directed that its role was not to make any policy determinations concerning the applicability of the AO Act to this group. Specifically, the committee was charged to

- evaluate the reliability (including representativeness, consistency, methods used) of the available information for establishing exposure; and
- address and place in context (qualitatively by comparison to established exposure guidelines) whether any documented residues represent potentially harmful exposure by characterizing the amounts available and the degree to which absorption might be expected.

The possible health effects associated with these exposures would be assumed to be those characterized in prior IOM Veterans and Agent Orange (VAO) reports and were not to be reassessed for this report.

THE COMMITTEE'S APPROACH

At its initial meeting, the committee decided to undertake several activities in three general areas in order to complete its tasks.

1. Organize the available information, identify gaps and inconsistencies, and endeavor to resolve such issues.

    - Screen for relevance and categorize the documents provided.
    - Gather information on existing health guidelines and their derivations.
    - Evaluate the sampling procedures and results.
    - Conduct a workshop to clarify issues and to obtain missing information.

2. Evaluate existing information and determine what interpretations regarding exposure were supported.

    - Consider various interpretations of the available data.
    - Review existing exposure estimation models.
    - Evaluate whether the detected AO residues could have reached the AF Reservists' bodies and then been absorbed.
    - Establish plausible magnitude of the AF Reservists' exposure.

3. In the context of existing guidelines for 2,3,7,8-tetrachlorodibenzo-*p*-dioxin (TCDD or dioxin) and dioxin-like compounds (the toxic contaminants of some of the herbicides sprayed in Vietnam), assess whether the magnitude of exposure supported by the existing information could plausibly be associated with adverse health effects during the time period when the AF Reservists were potentially exposed.

How the committee went about performing these activities is elaborated in Chapter 1, while the results of those efforts are summarized below.

THE AVAILABLE INFORMATION

The committee evaluated an assortment of documents submitted by the VA, veterans, and other interested parties, and collected relevant data from published journal articles and technical guidelines developed by authoritative organizations. The VA provided the committee with the sparse sampling data available for the C-123 aircraft and all relevant associated background information on the history of the planes' use and sampling, plus several military interpretations of these data and an extensive set of possibly pertinent documents. The C-123 Veterans Association and other interested parties provided historical records, personal accounts of service aboard C-123s, procedure manuals, aircraft logs, and some flight information from Air Squadrons and AF Reserve bases. The committee obtained a considerable amount of additional information, particularly on technical matters and guidelines from authoritative bodies, from the peer-reviewed literature. It also scanned a considerable amount of non-peer-reviewed material available on the Internet for clues that might lead to more definitive sources. The committee also held a public workshop to gather additional information and to hear from veterans and veterans' service organizations, representatives from the VA, researchers, and other interested parties.

Some fundamental information about the exposure of the AF Reservists was either not recoverable at all or the content provided by various sources could not be reconciled. For instance, considerable effort has failed to establish exactly how many C-123s the military had in Vietnam; how many of them for spraying insecticides; how many were used for spraying herbicides (the ones referred to in this report as ORH C-123s), how many were returned to the United States, how many ORH C-123s and how many C-123s that had not been in Vietnam were allocated to the various reserve units; and how many AF Reservists possibly worked in ORH C-123s.

As would be expected as a consequence of photolysis with exposure to sunlight and non-containment of volatilized chemicals, when several C-123s were finally sampled, their exteriors were not demonstrably contaminated with residues of TCDD or the herbicides sprayed in Vietnam. Only a very small number of samples for measurement of TCDD and the herbicides in AO were taken from the interior surfaces and from the air in a small number of the ORH C-123s flown by the AF Reservists (see Table S-1 for an inventory).

At the time of the 1979 sampling, methods of TCDD analysis were not readily available and had limited sensitivity, but TCDD is generally recognized as being more toxic than the herbicides, which are also less persistent than this contaminant. The committee, therefore, considered TCDD to be the component of the ORH-derived chemicals most relevant for assessing health risk. The short

TABLE S-1 Summary of Interior Sampling Efforts Conducted on C-123 Aircraft Previously Used to Spray Herbicides in Operation Ranch Hand

	Surface		Air	
Year	TCDD	2,4-D 2,4,5-T	TCDD	2,4-D 2,4,5-T
1979		2 from A		3 from A
1994	3 from A			
1995	5 from A			
1996	2 from unknown (not usable)	2 each from B, C + 10 more		
2009	7 from B, 9 from C	7 from B, 9 from C	1 each from B + C	1 each from B + C

NOTES: Number of interior samples taken from specific C-123s with documented use in Operation Ranch Hand.
C-123 tail numbers: A = #56-4362 (i.e., "Patches"); B = #55-4532; C = #55-4571.

periods over which the two TCDD air samples were gathered make them of questionable reliability, so the committee focused its qualitative assessment on the interior TCDD wipe samples collected from a total of three ORH C-123s. The two interior surface samples without information on area sampled could not be converted into usable results. The 24 usable measurements are graphed in Figure S-1.

EVALUATION AND INTERPRETATION

The long delay between when the exposures occurred (1972–1982) and when the measurements were made (1979 for herbicides only and not until the mid-1990s and 2009 for TCDD) is a serious limitation of the sampling data. Over this long period, degradation and loss processes were occurring to an unknown extent, so the levels when the Reservists were exposed would have been at least as high as the measurements made later. The lack of knowledge about decreases in TCDD and herbicide concentrations between the AF Reservists' time in the C-123s and later sampling precludes any attempts to make adjustments for a predicted decay in concentration. The delay before sampling contributes additional uncertainty to any quantitative estimates made of exposure, while very likely biasing the results toward underestimates. There also is uncertainty about the fraction of the C-123s worked in by the AF Reservists that had actually been used to spray herbicides in ORH, in addition to very incomplete knowledge of the AF Reservists' profiles of work that would be needed to estimate the contact rate, frequency, and time in quantitative modeling.

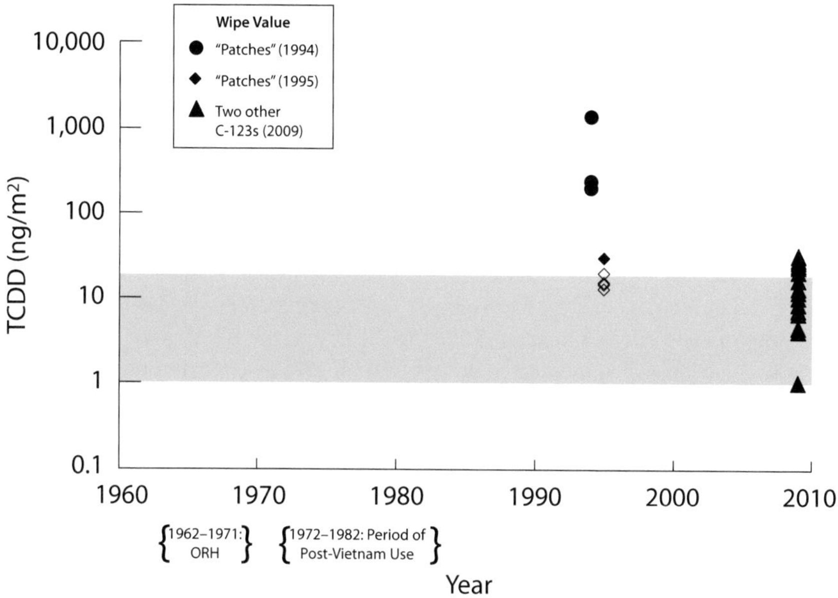

FIGURE S-1 Existing TCDD surface concentrations in relation to interior wipe samples.
NOTES: TCDD surface concentrations obtained from the total of 24 wipe samples from the interiors of ORH C-123 aircraft by year. The horizontal band represents the 1–25 ng/m^2 range of existing surface guidelines for TCDD.
Clear points represent non-detect samples plotted at their detection limit. The concentration of TCDD in four samples gathered from "Patches" in 1994 were below their limits of detection, which in turn were not sensitive enough to evaluate whether or not the samples' concentrations were less than 1 ng/m^2 (below the range of concern).

The committee assessed arguments presented in previous interpretations of the available information on AO contamination of the C-123s used by the AF Reservists from 1972–1982. It noted that those from in the military or associated with the VA tended to minimize the possibility of an increased risk of exposure and adverse health outcomes among the AF Reservists. A recurrent theme in these assertions was that dry AO residues containing TCDD detected on interior surfaces of ORH C-123s long after the planes returned from Vietnam could not have moved from the surfaces and thus were unable to complete transfer to the "outer boundary of a human" to constitute exposure as defined by the US Army's Center for Health Promotion and Preventive Medicine. The committee notes emphatically: it is now accepted in the field of exposure science that the physicochemical properties of semi-volatile organic compounds (SVOCs) like TCDD keep them in dynamic flux toward equilibrium in enclosed spaces among the various phases present (liquid, gas in air, airborne particles, dust on surfaces, residues or films on surfaces).

The committee explored the range of exposure estimates generated when plausible scenarios were used as input for the various exposure models proposed in the reviewed literature for estimating potential exposure from the available data. To put such findings in context, they were compared to existing guidelines for TCDD exposure within enclosed settings. When making such comparisons, the committee was contrasting the range of values it had adopted as being realistic for the AF Reservists for the variables in the models (such as frequency and duration of exposure in the contaminated environment, contact with surfaces, and breathing rates) to the extreme values assumed for the office worker population for which the guidelines had been developed (for example, 30 or 40 years working in a contaminated office). Compared to office workers, the AF Reservists' engaged in more vigorous movements and activities with greater exposure potential (such as having more contact with additional surfaces, sitting on the floor of the aircraft, having limited or no access to lavatory facilities, eating in the contaminated area), which suggests they would have experienced higher exposure from inadvertent ingestion and dermal pathways than office workers. On the other hand, the number of hours and years that the AF Reservists worked in the aircraft were less than what was assumed in establishing guidelines for the office workers. Setting aside efforts to equate the quite uncertain work profiles of the AF Reservists to the extreme work patterns assumed when deriving guidelines intended to apply to all office workers, the committee regarded the assembled existing guidelines for surface loading, which ranged from 1 to 25 ng/m^2, as a rough basis for assessing the set of sampling measurements presented in Figure S-1.

The committee found that none of the exposure models considered incorporated the full spectrum of plausible exposure routes. As a result, these exposure models would generate underestimates of actual exposure when "best" or plausible exposure estimates were sought. Similarly, by overlooking plausible routes of exposure, existing guidelines may overstate the level of protection their values actually provide. Another variant of this problem arose in a 2009 report prepared for Hill Air Force Base that derived screening guidelines for TCDD and the phenoxy herbicides that were intended to take into account both oral and dermal routes of exposure; the committee found that use of an erroneous formula had resulted in screening standards purportedly for oral and dermal exposure that effectively discounted the more sensitive dermal route. This standard was used in several subsequent interpretations of the C-123 TCDD sampling data under the assumption that it was more protective or stringent than was the case, thereby understating associated health risks.

In exploring exposure estimates consistent with the observed sampling results, the committee considered plausible, rather than "worst-case," scenarios. Having considered a variety of approaches for interpreting the available data and having established the intrinsic weaknesses of those data for quantitative exposure estimation, the committee was unable to determine which, if any, of the various models and exposure scenarios it investigated were most representative of the experiences of the AF Reservists. The committee observed, however, that, under at least some of the scenarios, all the quantitative models generated exposure estimates for the C-123 personnel that were larger than what screening guidelines deemed to be "acceptably" safe.

When putting its perceptions of the available surface sampling measurements in context by comparison to existing protective guidelines, however, the committee did proceed in accord with the public health practice, often referred to as the "precautionary principle," that seeks to identify possibly dangerous situations and to provide warning about health before, or at levels below where a problem is evident. Factors contributing to uncertainty discussed in this report (perhaps most importantly the long delay between when the activities leading to possible exposure occurred and sampling, and the guidelines' failure to account for the extent of dermal absorption) would mean that the measured TCDD surface levels would in all likelihood understate the risk of adverse health effects to which the AF Reservists actually had been exposed.

Because these individually uncertain perspectives on the situation consistently supported the possibility of health risks, the committee concluded that the available information supports the expectation that the health of some of the personnel was adversely affected by their service in the C-123s that had earlier been used to spray herbicides in Vietnam.

THE COMMITTEE'S FINDINGS

Assessment of Available Information

- The sampling efforts were not designed to quantitatively assess the potential exposure to the AF Reservists.
- The fact that TCDD sampling was not contemporaneous with the period when the AF Reservists experienced exposure complicates efforts to use the results to assess the possibility that harm to their health may have occurred.
- Sampling and analysis methods used over the various sampling periods apparently were not uniform, but the methodologies were not fully described. Aside from the air samples which were collected using inappropriate methods, however, the committee did not find information to invalidate any of the reported measurement data.
- Considerable nonuniformity in the distribution of contamination throughout the interior of "Patches" and differences in sampling procedures may have contributed to the inconsistencies noted between the sampling results in 1994 and 1995.
- Detailed, reliable information is not available on the activities of aircrews and maintenance personnel inside these airplanes (e.g., time spent in

planes, contacts with surfaces, use of protective equipment, etc.) and very little information is available on the use of specific aircraft.

Interpretation of Available Information

- The limitations of the available information make the data inadequate for deriving definitive quantitative estimates of exposure, but they are sufficient for a screening level of analysis.
- The interiors of the C-123s that had sprayed herbicides in Vietnam and were later used by the AF Reservists had AO and TCDD contamination persisting long after their use by the AF Reserve personnel.
- Understanding of the physical and chemical characteristics of SVOCs like TCDD establishes that they would not have been immobilized on surfaces, so residues were available for transfer by dermal contact, inhalation, and ingestion. The AF Reservists serving in the contaminated C-123s, therefore, experienced some degree of exposure to TCDD and herbicides through multiple routes when working in ORH C-123s.
- How representative the very limited number of TCDD samples gathered from the ORH C-123s are of the TCDD distribution throughout their interiors is uncertain, but, in the absence of definitive information to the contrary, the committee assumed that the three ORH C-123s sampled were representative of the entire fleet.
- There is no definitive information on the rate of degradation of TCDD on interior surfaces of the aircraft in the decades after their use in ORH. Without adjustment for reductions in the contamination over time, estimates of TCDD exposures to the AF Reservists based on samples taken from the C-123s in the mid-1990s and in 2009 could therefore underestimate their actual exposures, quite possibly markedly. Therefore, the measurements resulting from interior surface sampling in 1994, 1995, and 2009 probably represent a lower bound on what average surface TCDD contamination might have been when AF Reservists worked in the planes.
- Because of issues concerning inadequate factoring of dermal absorption into the development of guidelines, the committee recognized that several of the guidelines referred to during its evaluation were likely not as protective as might be supposed.
- The committee did not find any of the existing contamination guidelines for TCDD that it reviewed or the three models as presented and parameterized in Lurker et al. (2014) to be a perfect match for the circumstances being evaluated, which (in addition to the committee charge to conduct a qualitative evaluation and the limitations of the available data) represents another impediment to quantitative estimation of the Reservists' exposures or risks.

- The committee did decide that the surface Toxicity Equivalency Quotient (TEQ) loading guidelines were most applicable to the AF Reservists' occupational situation. It is the committee's judgment that comparing the unadjusted surface measurements from the ORH C-123s to the existing guidelines for surface loading provides the most valid qualitative means of evaluating the degree to which these results supported exposures safely less than international regulatory standards.
- The existing guidelines for TEQs on interior surfaces ranged from 1 to 25 ng/m^2, a zone in which sampling measurements reach a level where further action would be appropriate.

Although the existing information is inadequate for estimating exposure with any degree of certainty, the committee was able to answer its charge to evaluate the reliability of the data and to qualitatively establish whether the documented residues represent potentially harmful exposures.

Based upon physicochemical principles, the committee rejected the idea that the dioxin residues detected on interior surfaces of the ORH C-123s were immobile and effectively inaccessible to the Reservists as a source of exposure. Accordingly, the committee states with confidence that the AF Reservists ***were exposed*** when working in the ORH C-123s and so ***experienced some increase in their risk*** of a variety of adverse responses. The committee has shown that ***results of the most relevant type of sampling*** (which were collected a very long time after the AF Reservists worked in the ORH C-123s) fall ***in or above*** the 1-to-25 ng/m^2 range specified as meriting cautionary consideration by international exposure guidelines.

Efforts to recover the work records of the AF Reservists have been unsuccessful. The committee surmises it is unlikely that any additional information will become available to establish more definitively the magnitude of exposures experienced by the AF Reservists.

1

Introduction

In 1991, Congress passed Public Law 102-4, the Agent Orange Act of 1991, which directed the Secretary of Veterans Affairs to contract with the National Academy of Sciences (NAS) to conduct an independent review of scientific information regarding the association, if any, between health outcomes and exposure to dioxin or other chemical compounds in the herbicides that were sprayed in Vietnam. According to that legislation, any "veteran who, during active military, naval, or air service, served in the Republic of Vietnam during the Vietnam era [January 9, 1962–May 7, 1975, for compensation purposes] . . . shall be presumed to have been exposed during such service to an herbicide agent" and "whenever the Secretary [of Veterans Affairs] determines . . . that a positive association exists between the exposure of humans to an herbicide agent and the occurrence of disease in humans, the Secretary shall prescribe regulations providing that a presumption of service connection is warranted." With the passage of time, the straightforward interpretation of this legislation—that a "Vietnam veteran" who contracts a disease that has been determined to be associated with herbicide exposure would be eligible for compensation benefits—has been subjected to a number of challenges. The presumption of exposure to herbicides has been extended to veterans who served in the Korean demilitarized zone any time between April 1, 1968, and August 1, 1971. Another dispute has surrounded the eligibility of naval veterans from the Vietnam era; resolution of this issue by the US Department of Veterans Affairs (VA) has been that individuals who served on ships when they operated on Vietnam's inland waterways (the Brown Water Navy) are considered eligible, whereas other era veterans (the Blue Water Navy) are eligible only if they can establish that they had "boots on the ground" in Vietnam. The current claims of the US Air Force (AF) Reservists who served in the United States in 1972–1982 on Fairchild UC-123 *Provider* aircraft that earlier had sprayed herbicides in Vietnam constitute yet another challenge concerning eligibility under the Agent Orange Act of 1991.

From 1972 to 1982, approximately 1,500–2,100 AF Reserve personnel trained and worked on UC-123 aircraft, of which about 30 formerly had been used to spray herbicides in Vietnam as part of Operation Ranch Hand (ORH) (USAF, 2009a,b; Young and Young, 2013a). ORH missions sprayed the herbicides picloram and cacodylic acid, and chemical formulations that contained the herbicides 2,4-dichlorophenoxyacetic acid (2,4-D) and 2,4,5-trichlorophenoxyacetic acid (2,4,5-T); 2,4,5-T contained 2,3,7,8-tetrachlorodibenzo-*p*-dioxin (TCDD or dioxin), an unintended contaminant that was later determined to be a human carcinogen. Results of air and wipe samples taken between 1979 and 2009 by the AF (or its contractors) from the aircraft formerly used in ORH (ORH C-123s) indicate that residual chemicals from the Agent Orange (AO) and other herbicides that were sprayed in Vietnam remained on the interior of some of the aircraft. In 2012, the USAF School of Aerospace Medicine conducted an exposure assessment to quantify the potential exposure to AO by the AF Reserve personnel or passengers who flew on the C-123 aircraft in the United States, and determined that AO exposures "were unlikely to have exceeded acceptable regulatory standards or to have predisposed persons . . . to experience future adverse outcomes" (USAF, 2012a).

The VA Office of Public Health interpreted these findings to mean that "the existing scientific studies and reports support a low probability that TCDD was biologically available in these aircraft. Therefore, the potential for exposure to TCDD from flying or working in contaminated C-123 aircraft years after the Vietnam War is unlikely to have occurred at levels that could affect health" (VA, 2014). Because of lingering concerns among AF Reserve personnel about the potential for adverse health outcomes as a result of their service aboard C-123 aircraft that were formerly used in Vietnam to spray defoliants, the VA requested that the Institute of Medicine (IOM) conduct a review of the available C-123 sampling data, compare the data to existing exposure safety guidelines, and make a determination about the potential for exposure to the residual chemicals by C-123 personnel and associated concerns regarding possible adverse health consequences.

CHARGE TO THE COMMITTEE

In early 2014, the VA contracted with the IOM to conduct a study to determine whether or not crew members who flew C-123 aircraft that had previously been used to spray herbicides in Vietnam, had exposures that could have been detrimental to their health. In response, the IOM assembled an expert committee (see Appendix C for the committee member biographies) to determine whether there had been exposures that could lead to excess risk of adverse health outcomes among AF Reserve personnel who flew in and/or maintained C-123 aircraft (outside of Vietnam) that had previously been used to spray AO in Vietnam. The committee was asked to

- evaluate the reliability (including representativeness, consistency, methods used) of the available information for establishing exposure; and
- address and place in context (qualitatively by comparison to established exposure guidelines) whether any documented residues represent potentially harmful exposure by characterizing the amounts available and the degree to which absorption might be expected.

The possible health effects were to be those characterized in prior IOM Veterans and Agent Orange (VAO) reports, and they were not to be reassessed for this report. VAO committees to date have found the information concerning the exposure of Vietnam veterans inadequate to establish dose–response relationships for individual health outcomes or to quantify the risk of a particular veteran experiencing any adverse effects from such exposures. In any event, the possibility of an increase in the risk of any adverse health condition is the outcome to be assessed in this report.

THE COMMITTEE'S APPROACH TO ITS CHARGE

One of the fundamental differences between this report and prior IOM reports that have focused on other veteran cohorts—Vietnam veterans, Blue Water Navy veterans, and so on—is in the existence of exposure data that are relevant to the population of interest. The primary focus of this committee's deliberations is on the results of air and wipe sampling data, collected between 1979 and 2009, from ORH C-123 aircraft that were used by the AF Reserve personnel between 1972 and 1982. These samples were analyzed for the phenoxy herbicides and the TCDD-contaminant of 2,4,5-T. Sampling data from 1979, 1994, 1996, and 2009—in the form of laboratory reports, internal USAF reports and memorandums, or data reports—were provided to the committee by the VA at the beginning of this effort. Additional sampling results from 1996 were transmitted from the VA to the committee after the IOM staff inquired about the existence of additional samples that were referred to in an article critique (Nieman, 2014) but not received by the committee. In reviewing all the available sampling data, the committee evaluated the sampling methods, laboratory procedures and protocols, and assumptions, to the extent that information in the documents permitted such assessment.

From among the materials provided by the VA, the committee reviewed independent interpretations of the USAF C-123 sampling data authored by entities associated with the military, representatives of the Agency for Toxic Substances and Disease Registry (ATSDR) and the National Institute of Environmental

Health Sciences (NIEHS), and several independent researchers. The committee also spent considerable time in evaluating a recently published paper by Lurker et al. (2014) that used the available C-123 sampling data to derive quantitative estimates of the exposure of the AF Reservists.

The committee held a public workshop to gather additional information and to hear from veterans and veterans service organizations, representatives of the VA, researchers, and other interested parties (see Appendix A for all open session agendas). This open session gave members of the committee an opportunity to learn more about the use of C-123s both in Vietnam and afterward by the AF Reserve personnel and related issues. Before the workshop, the committee distributed a list of questions to workshop participants that focused on issues pertaining to post-Vietnam handling and use of the C-123s by the AF Reserve personnel, collection and analysis of air and wipe samples from ORH C-123s, modeling efforts that used the existing sampling data, and interpretations of resulting exposure estimates. Participants were asked to address these questions in writing and during their presentations to the committee, and their submissions and later discussions formed the basis of in-depth panel discussions and question and answer sessions during the public workshop.

In fulfilling its charge, the committee evaluated numerous documents submitted by the VA, the C-123 Veterans Association, individual veterans, and other interested parties; and it collected relevant data from published journal articles and technical guidelines derived by authoritative international bodies, such as the World Health Organization and the US Environmental Protection Agency. In addition to information pertaining to the sampling data, the VA gave the committee an extensive collection of possibly pertinent documents, including published papers, technical exposure guidelines, internal AF memos and reports, National Institute for Occupational Safety and Health (NIOSH) reports, early exposure reports from the NAS, and photographs. The C-123 Veterans Association and other interested parties provided historical records and personal accounts of their service aboard C-123s during their AF Reserve careers, C-123 procedure manuals, examples of aircraft logs, and flight information from air squadrons and the AF Reserve bases. The committee has cited these materials extensively in its report and has provided copies of the referenced materials to the Public Access Records Office of the National Academies. They can be accessed by emailing PARO@nas.edu or calling 202-334-3543.

The committee faced several challenges during the course of its deliberations. Much of the information that the committee reviewed was anecdotal in nature and so was difficult to verify with historical documentation. A great deal of the historical information provided to the committee was in the form of memorandums and other personal correspondence, so it was difficult or impossible to acquire more specific information, especially that related to details of the AF sampling efforts, such as sampling strategies, collection procedures, and laboratory testing or analysis or to work profiles for the AF Reservists. The committee evaluated all of the available documentation with some skepticism, inasmuch as the likelihood of bias could not be completely ruled out.

ORGANIZATION OF THE REPORT

The remainder of this report is organized into four more chapters and three appendixes. Chapter 2 contains basic background information on the chemical properties of TCDD and a compilation of health guidelines for this compound and consideration of their applicability to the experience of the AF Reservists for use in putting the available sampling data in context. Information about the use of C-123 aircraft in Vietnam and their later use by AF Reserve personnel in the United States and the collection of air and wipe samples from some of these aircraft between 1979 and 2009, are discussed in Chapter 3. Chapter 4 reviews interpretations of those sampling results by the AF and individuals in the dioxin research community. It also evaluates exposure models applied to the C-123 sampling data in Lurker et al. (2014), addresses the plausibility that residues measured on internal surfaces could have been absorbed into the bodies of the AF Reservists, and discusses the committee's thoughts about how the available information relates to international exposure guidelines. A compilation of the committee's findings is presented in Chapter 5.

2

TCDD: Physicochemical Properties and Health Guidelines

Of the components and contaminants of the several herbicides used by the US military in Vietnam, 2,3,7,8-tetrachlorodibenzo-*p*-dioxin (TCDD) stands out as having the greatest toxic potency. It was an unintended contaminant of 2,4,5-trichlorophenoxyacetic acid (2,4,5-T), one of the phenoxy herbicides comprising Agent Orange (AO) and also Agents Pink, Green, and Purple (IOM, 2014). TCDD, or dioxin, is the most toxic of the polychlorinated dibenzo-*p*-dioxin (PCDD), dibenzofuran (PCDF), and biphenyl (PCB) congeners. Several of the PCDD, PCDF, and PCB congeners share TCDD's major mechanism of action in producing several adverse health conditions by binding to the aryl hydrocarbon receptor (AHR), but at a fraction of its potency. Toxic Equivalency Factors (TEFs), where the TEF of TCDD has a value of one, have been assigned to these congeners providing the basis for a summary metric that expresses the total "dioxin-like activity" in a mixture of chemicals, referred to as its Toxicity Equivalency Quotient (TEQ). The exceptionally high proportion of TEQs accounted for by TCDD itself in AO formulations (compared to other TCDD-containing mixtures) can serve as a chemical "signature" of these herbicides used by the military in Vietnam. After the Vietnam War, analyses of residual herbicide stocks found that contamination by the TCDD congener specifically ranged from less than 0.05 parts per million (ppm) up to almost 50 ppm, averaging 2–3 ppm (NRC, 1974; Young et al., 1978). Consequently, the TCDD contaminant of AO has been regarded as the primary reason for health concerns associated with exposure to the herbicides used in Vietnam, and so it is the committee's focus.

The committee reviewed those physical and chemical properties of TCDD that would influence its persistence in the C-123s that had been used in ORH, its availability for contacting the US Air Force (AF) Reservists when they worked inside these planes, and its presence in samples gathered considerably later. To establish a standard for putting the Reservists' exposures in context, the committee assembled existing health exposure guidelines for TCDD and considered the assumptions underlying them. These topics are discussed in this chapter.

PHYSICOCHEMICAL PROPERTIES OF TCDD IN THE INDOOR ENVIRONMENT

2,3,7,8-TCDD is a persistent organic pollutant and stable in the environment (EPA, 1992; IOM, 2011). It has very low water solubility and is typically removed from water and soil surfaces by photolysis and volatilization. The photolysis half-life at the water's surface has been estimated to range from 21 hours in summer to 118 hours in winter. The volatilization half-life from the water column of an environmental pond has been estimated to be 46 days; however, when the effects of adsorption to sediment are considered, the volatilization model predicts an overall volatilization removal half-life of over 50 years. Photodegradation on terrestrial surfaces may be an important transformation process. Volatilization from soil surfaces during warm conditions may be a major removal mechanism. The persistence half-life of TCDD on soil surfaces may vary from less than 1 year to 3 years, but half-lives in soil interiors may be as long as 12 years. Photodegradation is responsible for removal of TCDD from many surfaces (Karch et al., 2004). This phenomenon would be largely responsible for the failure to detect TCDD on the exteriors of the C-123s, but it would not be a major function on the aircraft's interiors, where flux toward equilibrium among media would be expected to dominate, with removal by airflow.

The physicochemical properties of a compound provide the scientific basis for determining how and to what extent a chemical may **come into contact with the "outer boundary of a human," the final step required for exposure to occur** as defined by the US Army's Center for Health Promotion and Preventive Medicine (CHPPM, 2009). Thirty-year-old residues deposited on a surface might be assumed to be effectively chemically inert as purported by the VA (http://www.publichealth.va.gov/exposures/agentorange/locations/residue-c123-aircraft/scientific-review.asp; accessed August 21, 2014) on the basis of reports from Young and Young (2012, 2013b). In fact, however, **semi-volatile organic compounds (SVOCs), such as TCDD, are in constant flux around equilibrium.**

Prior to reviewing past interpretations of the available sampling data, it is worthwhile to explore the theoretical distribution of TCDD and other SVOCs in the indoor environment and relate this to the exposure potential for AF Reserve personnel who served on C-123s that had formerly sprayed defoliants in Vietnam. The committee subscribes to the concepts related to fugacity as described in Weschler and Nazaroff (2008) that provide a holistic and dynamic view of multimedia transfer of these chemicals. These concepts can be summarized as follows:

1. Equilibrium partitioning of SVOCs between liquids, gas-phase air, airborne particles, dust on surfaces, residues or films on surfaces, and humans, governs the fate and transport of these chemicals.
2. With a saturation vapor pressure of 3.9×10^{-12} atm, TCDD is classified as an SVOC (where SVOCs are defined as having vapor pressures between 10^{-14} and 10^{-4}).
3. Indoor surfaces have films (i.e., a mix of organics, inorganic ions, water, and particles) that interact with gas-phase SVOCs; it is likely that these films play a larger role than bare surfaces in transport and exposure.
4. Most indoor environments are dynamic, resulting in exchanges in mass across compartments that are nearly continuously in flux.

From these concepts we can assume that a satisfactory sampling scheme would involve multiple media types (such as air, residue or films, and dust). If it is present in one medium, an SVOC like TCDD would be expected to partition into other environmental compartments, as has been demonstrated for the SVOCs phthalates inside a stainless steel chamber (Liang and Xu, 2014). Processes (such as ventilation and cleaning) may remove chemicals from one compartment; however, if a reservoir exists, over time dynamic partitioning will likely replenish the chemical to a state of equilibrium.

The nature of films that can harbor organic chemicals on nonporous surfaces has been established on glass (Liu et al., 2003) and on metal surfaces (Wallace et al., 2014). Together, these articles demonstrate that, in environments where there are organic materials, an organic film will coat the types of inert surfaces (i.e., metals, glass, and plastic) that are found inside aircraft. The thickness of the film will depend on the type of organic material present (for example, skin oils and greases used or present in aircraft), temperature, and time since the surface was cleaned by some process such as heating, wiping, or solvent treatment. The organic film then serves as both a source from which SVOCs will emanate and a medium into which they will be absorbed in an equilibrium process.

Exposures to herbicide and TCDD residues in the C-123s could occur via three pathways: dermal, inhalation, and ingestion. The characterization of external exposure for each pathway needs to incorporate the concentrations in the relevant media that reach a body boundary, the frequency of that contact, and the duration of the contact. Those data, when coupled with the transference or uptake into the body can provide an internal exposure or dose.

The principle that SVOCs (including TCDD) migrate "downhill" along thermodynamic gradients is generally accepted by physical chemists (Mackay, 2001) and the exposure assessment community (Bennett and Furtaw, 2004; Weschler and Nazaroff, 2008). **The former Operation Ranch Hand (ORH) C-123s were contaminated with TCDD, and the AF Reservists were "downhill" when inside the planes. As a consequence, they would have been exposed to TCDD, but the magnitude of the doses they received are quite uncertain.**

EXISTING HEALTH GUIDELINES FOR TCDD EXPOSURE

Screening guidelines are derived as standards for assessing whether further action is appropriate for a particular situation because of the ***possibility*** of adverse health outcomes of any sort in a ***group***. They are not meant to predict the number of adverse events that will be observed, but are intended to be ***protective*** of a broad range of activities and sensitivities.

Although TCDD is a naturally occurring combustion product, it has never been an intended product of any industrial process. Consequently, although dioxin guidelines have been developed by expert bodies such as the US Environmental Protection Agency (EPA) and the World Health Organization (WHO) in an effort to protect the general population from harmful levels of intake from environmental sources, TCDD itself has not been a common target of occupational regulation.

In the past, PCBs were purposefully handled in industrial settings and became of increased concern as the adverse consequences of dispersed and combusted PCBs following transformer fires came to light. This necessitated development of re-entry standards for fire-impacted buildings. The recognition that most of the toxicity of PCBs and also furans results from specific congeners that share the AH-receptor mechanism of action with TCDD with a lower degree of potency has permitted development of a unified measure of toxic potency for dioxins, PCBs, and furans. Exposure standards for these chemicals have been set in terms of TEQs, which are the summed TEFs weighted by the measured amount of their associated congener in a particular analyzed sample.

Various agencies and other groups have proposed guidelines for exposure to TCDD and dioxin-like chemicals through different routes. The recommended surface and air concentrations are guidelines for total intake. A surface contamination guideline assumes that the surface is the source of direct dermal exposure and possibly indirect ingestion and inhalation uptake that would provide a specified total intake, while a TCDD air guideline assumes that air is the sole source of TCDD. When there are multiple sources of exposure, the allowable uptakes from surfaces and from air need to be modified so that the corresponding guideline for total uptake is not exceeded.

All of the TCDD guidelines in Table 2-1 are for a weighted sum of different congeners and are expressed in terms of TEQs. Results in terms of TEQs were not presented for all the interior C-123 samples but, as demonstrated in the 1994 sampling of "Patches" (USAF, 1994), the vast majority of TEQs measured in samples from C-123 aircraft are derived from their TCDD content alone, as is characteristic of exposures derived from AO. As a result, **exposure limits in terms of TEQs provide an appropriate standard for comparison with TCDD samples drawn from the interior of the C-123 aircraft that had sprayed herbicides in Vietnam.**

Like estimation of the amount of exposure experienced, estimation of the dose–response portion of the risk assessment calculations entails many sources of

TABLE 2-1 Available Guidelines Concerning Exposure to TCDD

Intended Application (Name)	Authority (Citation)	Guideline (TEQs) Daily Intake (pg/kg-d)	Air Concentration (pg/m^3)	Surface Loading (ng/m^2)
Occupational Air Standard				
(TLV)	Germany (German MAK-Wert, 1999)		10	
Building Re-entry				
	National Research Council (NRC, 1988)	2	10	25
	NRC Table 2			
	California (Gravitz et al., 1983)	1.8–23	10	3
	State of New York (Kim and Hawley, 1985)	2	10	25
	New Mexico (Melius, 1985)		2	1
	Louisiana (NRC, 1988)	26–650	1.5	25
	Technical Guide 312 (CHPPM, 2009)			3.5
	World Trade Center Working Group (WTC, 2003)		1	2
General Public				
(MRL)	ATSDR (1998)	200		
(MRL)	ATSDR (1998)	20		
(MRL)	ATSDR (1998)	1		

Lifetime Risk	Population Targeted by Guideline	Exposure Duration	Routes Included in Guideline (source-mode of entry)
4×10^{-4} to 4×10^{-3} cancer	70-kg adult	40-yr working lifetime	Air: inhalation
< 2×10^{-4} cancer	Adult office worker	30 yrs	Air: inhalation; Surface residues: ingestion, inhalation
1×10^{-6} to 5×10^{-5} cancer	65–70-kg adult office worker	Working lifetime	
9×10^{-8} to 2×10^{-4} cancer	50-kg adult office worker	250 days/yr, 30 years	Air: inhalation; Surface residues: ingestion, inhalation
< 1×10^{-6} cancer	Adult office worker	Working lifetime	
	65-kg adult office worker	Working lifetime	
1×10^{-6} cancer	Long-term office workers		Surface residues: ingestion, dermal, and inhalation
1×10^{-4} cancer	70-kg adult	Residence for 30 yrs, 365 days/yr, 24 hr/day	Air: inhalation; Settled dust: ingestion, dermal
	General public	Acute(< 15 days)	Oral
	General public	Intermediate (15–364 days)	Oral
	General public	Chronic (≥ 365 days)	Oral

continued

TABLE 2-1 Continued

		Guideline (TEQs)		
Intended Application (Name)	Authority (Citation)	Daily Intake (pg/kg-d)	Air Concentration (pg/m³)	Surface Loading (ng/m²)
(PTI)	Australia and Canada (WHO, 2002a,b)	70 pg/kg-*month* TEQ for dioxins, furans, and PCBs ~ 2.3 pg/kg-d for TCDD		
(TDI)	Japan (Japanese EA, 1999)	4		
(TDI)	Denmark, Finland, Sweden (Johansson and Hanberg, 2000)	5		
(TDI)	Netherlands (RIVM, 2001)	1–4		
(PTI)	European Commission's Scientific Committee on Food (EC, 2001)	14 pg/kg-*week* TEQ for dioxins, furans, and PCBs ~ 2 pg/kg-d for TCDD		
(TDI)	JECFA (WHO, 2002a,b)	~ 1 pg/kg-d		
(TDI)	UK Environment Agency (UKEA, 2009)	2 [retained standard set in 2003]		
(CSF)	US EPA (EPA, 2000)	1.5×10^{-4} $(pg/kg\text{-}d)^{-1}$		
(RfD)	US EPA (EPA, 2012)	0.7	40	
	California EPA (1999)	10		

NOTES: ADI, acceptable daily intake; ATSDR, Agency for Toxic Substances and Disease Registry; CSF, cancer slope factor; EPA, Environmental Protection Agency; JECFA, Joint FAO/WHO Expert Committee on Food Additives; kg-time, body weight of exposed individual over specified time period; LADD, lifetime average daily dose; LOAEL, lowest-observed-adverse-effect level; MRL, minimal risk level (daily human exposure that is likely to be without appreciable risk of adverse, noncancer effects over a specified duration of exposure—ATSDR); NOEL, no-observed-effect level; NRC, National Research Council; OEL, occupational exposure limit; PTI, provisional tolerable intake; RfD, reference dose (estimate with uncertainty spanning about an order of magnitude of a daily exposure likely to be without appreciable risk of deleterious noncancer effects during a lifetime); TDI, tolerable daily intake; TLV, threshold limit value; TWA, time-weighted average.

Lifetime Risk	Population Targeted by Guideline	Exposure Duration	Routes Included in Guideline (source-mode of entry)
	General public	Cumulative over extended period	Oral
	General public	Chronic	Oral
	General public	Chronic	Oral
	General public	Lifetime	Oral
	General public	Chronic	Oral
	General public	Chronic	Oral
	General public	Lifetime	Oral and inhalation
	General public	Continuous exposure over lifetime	Oral
	General public	Lifetime	

uncertainty. Although determination of an agent's toxicity to humans is the objective, the numerous uncontrolled factors involved in epidemiologic results (which underlie conclusions concerning association reached in the IOM's Veterans and Agent Orange series) dictate that results of laboratory experiments are most often used. The estimates of toxic potency underlying the guidelines referred to by the committee in assessing concern about the exposure of the AF Reservists who used C-123s that had sprayed herbicides in Vietnam have been derived from controlled animal studies. TCDD guidelines based on noncancer outcomes most often have been based on developmental effects, but a reduction in semen quality among young men exposed during the Seveso industrial accident (Moccarelli et al., 2008) was a determining factor in the noncancer reference dose (RfD) derived in a decades-long process (EPA, 2012).

For cancer outcomes (which are recognized among the adverse health effects associated with TCDD), the once generally accepted assumption of low-dose linearity dictates that some increase in risk is associated with any exposure—down to infinitesimal amounts that would be inconsequential. The resulting guideline, which is intended to protect against the occurrence of any cancer, will generally result in a lower concentration of the substance being regarded as safe than would be determined for a noncancer endpoint. For noncancer adverse effects (several of which are also on TCDD's generally accepted list of adverse outcomes), it has been thought that there is some level of exposure below which no toxic response would occur. It is now thought that such "threshold" dose–response models may also be applicable to certain mechanisms of toxicity that contribute to carcinogenesis. TCDD's AHR-mediated mode of biological activity, shared by other dioxin-like chemicals, appears to fit in this category. Small increments in exposure in a "threshold" situation do not pose a health threat if total exposure to agents with the mechanism of action in question is well below the estimated point of inflection in the dose–response curve. However, when "background" exposure experienced by the general public is still very close to "tolerable" daily intakes (TDIs in Table 2-1), a modest increment in exposure from an additional source can move an individual's total up to a level at which adverse effects are plausible.

The TCDD exposure guidelines (see Table 2-1) are of three types:

- those expressed in terms of daily TCDD intake (from all routes) per body weight (pg/kg-d),
- those expressed as an air concentration (pg/m^3), and
- those expressed in terms of surface contamination (ng/m^2).

Most of these surface contamination and air guidelines were derived for protection of office workers working in TCDD-contaminated buildings, and utilize exposure scenarios and assumptions pertaining to work practices of office workers, such as breathing rates, rate of contact of hands and arms with contaminated surfaces, percent of contaminant transferred to hands or arms after surface contact, etc. Each of the guidelines involves assumptions intended to ensure that keeping surface concentrations below the guideline would protect the health of a group. These health-protective assumptions increase the likelihood that, even if the guideline were exceeded, there may be no observable health effect in any individual in a population at risk. Screening levels are developed as a preliminary means of establishing whether health risks are sufficiently plausible that further investigation is needed, but for ORH C-123s and AF Reservists the information at hand is all there will ever be for decision making.

Guidelines developed for protection of the general public from exposure to TCDD and dioxin-like chemicals (focused on ingestion of food that has incorporated environmental contamination) are not directly applicable to evaluating the occupational exposures of the AF Reservists. They are, however, of interest in providing insight into cumulative lifetime intakes regarded by expert bodies such as EPA, the Agency for Toxic Substances and Disease Registry, and WHO, as falling at the borderline of acceptable. The committee found that, although no guideline was a perfect match for the experience of the AF Reservists, **the re-entry standards expressed in terms of surface loading are most applicable** for this situation.

Because fires involving PCB-containing equipment can release TCDD and PCB-related combustion products into the environment in toxicologically relevant concentrations, such fires are the basis for numerous federal and state regulatory and other actions designed to reduce human harm. EPA's "Transformer Rule" under Toxic Substance Control Act (40 Code of Federal Regulations, Part 761), for example, is a requirement to reduce hazards associated with combustion by-products or contaminants of PCBs in the transformers.

In 1988, the National Research Council's (NRC's) Committee on Toxicology, organized a Subcommittee on Dioxin that provided recommendations regarding acceptable contamination concentrations for TCDD to protect worker health upon re-entry into an office building after a transformer fire (NRC, 1988). At the time of the NRC report, four states (California, Louisiana, New Mexico, and New York) had TCDD surface concentration guidelines for worker re-entry after transformer fires in office buildings (see Table 2-1). For example, the NRC Subcommittee considered the recommended exposure guidelines put forth by the New York State Department of Health's risk assessment (Kim and Hawley, 1985) to be adequate for protecting long-term office workers from the harmful effects of dioxin. The New York guidelines were derived in part with a no-observed-effect level (NOEL)-safety factor approach, giving an assumed negligible likelihood of non-cancer health effects in humans. The TCDD guidelines of 10 pg/m^3 in air and 25 ng/m^2 on surfaces correspond to a 2 pg/kg allowable daily intake over a 30 year exposure period for a 50-kg office worker. The upper bound on lifetime cancer risk associated with the New York TCDD guidelines is 2×10^{-4}.

In Technical Guide 312 (TG 312) the Army Center for Health Promotion and Preventive Medicine (CHPPM, 2009) derives TCDD surface wipe screening levels (SWSLs) for long-term office workers. The screening level assumes exposure to contaminated surfaces through dermal contact and absorption, incidental ingestion by hand-to-mouth behaviors, and inhalation through breathing resuspended particulates. The upper bound cancer risk is set to 1×10^{-6} for a 70-kg office worker over a 10-year exposure duration. Environmental samples with concentrations above the 3.5 ng/m^2 SWSL for TCDD would be an indication for a more thorough health risk assessment for the site with more specific exposure parameters. A comparison of observed surface concentrations to the calculated TG 312 guidelines does not definitively distinguish between "safe and unsafe" environmental conditions, nor is an exceedance an "absolute predictor" of adverse health effects. Another military surface loading guideline was found in an AF interpretation of the sampling data (USAF, 2009b). It was said to be 22 ng/m^2, but should have been 1.1 ng/m^2 if it had correctly factored in the more sensitive dermal pathway as it was alleged to do (see discussion of Table 4-1).

In addition, after identifying dioxin as one of six contaminants of potential concern, the World Trade Center Indoor Air Task Force Working Group (WTC, 2003) went on to establish residential re-entry guidelines for each of these substances. To protect against a cancer risk of 10^{-4} for 70-kg adults living in a residence fulltime for 30 years, guidelines of 1 pg/m^3 indoor air was set for inhalation and 2 ng/m^2 in settled dust for dermal absorption and ingestion.

The guidelines for surface loading seem to be most applicable to the occupational situation this committee is evaluating. Also, almost all the usable TCDD sampling results happen to be measurements from surface wipes. **These screening guidelines in TEQs for surface loading range from 1 to 25 ng/m^2,** including the 3.5 ng/m^2 derived by CHPPM and the 22 ng/m^2 (or more correctly, 1.1 ng/m^2) guideline from the 2009 AF report. It is interesting to note the trend in these guidelines toward increasing stringency with the passage of time, a larger body of epidemiologic and experimental results, and improving understanding of the underlying biologic processes.

3

Air Force Use of the C-123 Provider: Background and Sampling Data

The Fairchild C-123 Provider is a short-range military assault aircraft used by the Air Force (AF) in Vietnam. Designed by the Chase Aircraft Company in New Jersey and built by Fairchild Industries in Hagerstown, Maryland, the C-123 was utilized in Vietnam for a range of tactical missions including transportation of military personnel and equipment, evacuation of wounded soldiers, and supply operations for advanced combat positions. This chapter provides background information about the use of C-123 Provider aircraft to spray herbicides in Vietnam and their subsequent use by the AF Reserve personnel in the United States. Descriptions of air and wipe samples collected from some of these aircraft between 1979 and 2009 by the US Air Force (USAF) are also presented.

USE OF C-123s IN VIETNAM

During the military conflict in Vietnam, one use of Fairchild UC-123 aircraft was flying defoliation missions to destroy enemy food supplies and to clear and expose enemy transportation and infiltration routes (IOM, 1994; Young, 2009; Young and Newton, 2004). "UC" was a designation given to C-123 aircraft that were equipped with spray apparatus. The UC-123s were estimated to have sprayed 88% of all herbicides used in Vietnam (AF Working Paper, 1979). Herbicide formulations used in defoliation efforts were composed of four compounds—2,4-dichlorophenoxyacetic acid (2,4-D), 2,4,5-trichlorophenoxyacetic acid (2,4,5-T), 4-amino-3,5,6-trichloropicolinic acid (picloram), and dimethylarsinic acid (cacodylic acid). An estimated 69 to 77 million liters of herbicides were sprayed over roughly 3.6 million acres in Vietnam between 1961 and 1971 (NRC, 1974; Stellman et al., 2003). The specific herbicide formulations (named for the band of color around each

55-gallon storage drum—Agents Pink, Green, Purple, Orange, White, and Blue), chemical composition, TCDD concentration, year used, and quantity sprayed are shown in Table 3-1.

Operation Ranch Hand

Historically, the approximately 1,300 AF personnel involved in the UC-123 fixed-wing aircraft spray activities in Vietnam between 1962 and 1971 (codenamed

TABLE 3-1 Military Use of Herbicides in Vietnam (1961–1971)

Code Name	Chemical Constituents[a]
Formulations with TCDD Contamination	
Pink	60% *n*-butyl ester, 40% isobutyl ester of 2,4,5-T
Green	*n*-butyl ester of 2,4,5-T
Purple	50% *n*-butyl ester of 2,4-D, 30% *n*-butyl ester of 2,4,5-T, 20% isobutyl ester of 2,4,5-T
Orange	50% *n*-butyl ester of 2,4-D, 50% *n*-butyl ester of 2,4,5-T
Orange II	50% *n*-butyl ester of 2,4-D, 50% isooctyl ester of 2,4,5-T
Formulations Without TCDD Contamination	
White	Acid weight basis: 21.2% triisopropanolamine salts of 2,4-D, 5.7% picloram
Blue powder	Cacodylic acid (dimethylarsinic acid) sodium cacodylate
Blue Aqueous solution	21% sodium cacodylate + cacodylic acid to yield at least 26% total acid equivalent by weight
Total, all formulations	—

NOTES: 2,4-D, 2,4-dichlorophenoxyacetic acid; 2,4,5-T, 2,4,5-trichlorophenoxyacetic acid; gal, gallon; L, liter; ppm, parts per million; TCDD, 2,3,7,8-tetrachlorodibenzo-*p*-dioxin; VAO, *Veterans and Agent Orange: Update 2012* (IOM, 2014).

Operation Ranch Hand [ORH]) have been considered among the most highly exposed workers to the chemicals that were in the defoliants. Defoliation spray missions were carried out by highly-trained three-person crews of male Ranch Hand (RH) personnel consisting of a pilot, copilot/navigator, and a spray equipment console operator. Personnel who provided primary maintenance for the ORH UC-123s

		Amount Sprayed	
TCDD Concentration	Years Used[a]	VAO Estimate[b]	Revised Estimate[a]
65.6 ppm	1961, 1965	464,817 L (122,792 gal)	50,312 L sprayed; 413,852 L more on procurement records
65.6 ppm	1961, 1965	31,071 L (8,208 gal)	31,026 L on procurement records
Up to 45 ppm	1962–1965	548,883 L (145,000 gal)	1,892,733 L
0.05–50 ppm (average, 1.98–2.99 ppm)	1965–1970	42,629,013 L (11,261,429 gal)	45,677,937 L (could include Agent Orange II)
0.05–50 ppm (average, 1.98–2.99 ppm)	After 1968	—	Unknown; at least 3,591,000 L shipped
None	1966–1971	19,860,108 L (5,246,502 gal)	20,556,525 L
None	1962–1964	—	25,650 L
None	1964–1971	4,255,952 L (1,124,307 gal)	4,715,731 L
	—	67,789,844 L (17,908,238 gal)	76,954,766 L (including procured)

[a] Based on Stellman et al., 2003.
[b] Based on data from MRI, 1967; NRC, 1974; Young and Reggiani, 1988.
SOURCES: Adapted from IOM, 2009, 2011.

were also potentially exposed to herbicides (AF Working Paper, 1979). Lurker et al. (2014) reported that the aircraft flew a total of almost 6,000 herbicide missions and became heavily contaminated with chemical residues during loading, maintenance, fueling, and while on missions. ORH crews had the potential for exposure when flying with the cockpit windows or rear cargo door open, flying through previously sprayed airspace, or by exposure to broken or malfunctioning spray lines or spillage from storage tanks. The extent of exposure of ORH ground crews or C-123 flight personnel in Vietnam has not been documented, but estimates of exposure based on days of exposure, percentage of skin exposed, the concentration of herbicide formulations, and serum TCDD concentrations, show that this population had the potential for even higher exposures than flight crews (Michalek et al., 1995).

USE OF C-123s AFTER THE VIETNAM CONFLICT

In 1970, the herbicide 2,4,5-T, which was included in the chemical formulations for Agent Orange (AO) (or Herbicide Orange), Agent Green, Agent Pink, and Agent Purple, was found to be contaminated with a byproduct of manufacturing, 2,3,7,8-tetrachlorodibenzo-*p*-dioxin (TCDD) or dioxin. Shortly thereafter, AO ORH missions were terminated after toxicologic studies found that TCDD caused congenital abnormalities in pregnant rodents (Courtney et al., 1970; Lindquist and Ullberg, 1971; Robinson et al., 2006). In late 1971, the White House issued an Executive Order, calling for the phasing out of all herbicide spray activities in Vietnam (AF Working Paper, 1979; Cecil, 1986). TCDD concentrations in AO samples taken after the Vietnam conflict varied from 0.05 parts per million (ppm) to nearly 66 ppm, with an average of 2–3 ppm (NRC, 1974, Young et al., 1978). At that time in the United States, TCDD contamination of 2,4,5-T could not exceed 0.5 ppm (NRC, 1974).

Between April 1969 and February 1972, 30–40 UC-123 aircraft used for ORH returned to the continental United States. Table B-1 in Appendix B lists these aircraft, as well as information on other ORH C-123s that did not return from Vietnam, compiled from Carter (2013), Alvin L. Young (personal communication, May 5, 2014), Young (2014), and Young and Young (2014a,b). Young and Young (2012, 2014a) report that of the former ORH aircraft, approximately 24 were distributed among AF Reserve units in the United States and thirteen were transferred to the Military Assistance Program (MAP), a program designed to sell aircraft to other nations for their military and domestic use.

All C-123s returning to the United States from Vietnam passed through the Military Aircraft Storage and Disposal Center (MASDC), which adjoins the Davis-Monthan Air Force Base (AFB) in Tucson, Arizona (Young and Young, 2014a,b). The MASDC facility operated as an aircraft storage, preservation, and maintenance facility for all the US Armed Forces. Typically aircraft arriving at this facility were reconditioned and returned to service; however, unsalvageable aircraft could be used for spare parts or target practice, transferred to other locations for museum displays, or smelted down into metal ingots and recycled (AMARG, 2014). Aircraft that arrived at this facility from Vietnam were stored for 3–6 months, during which time the spray tanks and booms were removed from the aircraft (Young and Young, 2014b).

Once spray equipment was removed from serviceable ORH aircraft, the C-123s were ferried to the Hayes Aircraft Facility at Napier Field, in Dothan, Alabama, to undergo reconditioning. The reconditioning process took between 3–6 months. Descriptions of the C-123 reconditioning process included cockpit standardization and engine repair; removal and replacement of all armor, seats, damaged flooring, and fuselage; instillation of new oxygen systems; industrial vacuuming; and internal and external cleaning and painting as appropriate for future use (Alvin L. Young, A.L. Young Consulting, Inc., personal communication, May 5, 2014; Young, 2014).

Written testimony provided by the C-123 Veterans Association to the committee, however, reported that the aircraft returning from Vietnam received only basic maintenance at a repair depot and needed extensive rehabilitation by maintenance personnel. The AF Reserve personnel reported that some C-123 aircraft arrived needing seats replaced, new litter stanchions, litter straps, first aid kits, matting, and in some aircraft, navigator stations. The exterior of some aircraft were patched but not repainted. The veteran's account stated that the AF Reserve crews worked to remove residue from the interior of the C-123 aircraft and exterior washing was undertaken with soap solutions applied with brushes and pressurized spray equipment (Carter, 2014a).

The efficacy of the reconditioning process or the AF Reservists' efforts in removing remnants of herbicides sprayed in ORH is at odds with the existing results from samples drawn many years later, which are the focus of this report.

Assignment of C-123s to AF Reserve Units

Once cleared from Napier Field, C-123 aircraft formerly used for ORH were assigned to AF Reserve units or sold overseas. The C-123s that remained in the United States were transferred to the 906th or 907th Tactical Airlift Groups (TAGs) located at the Lockbourne/Rickenbacker AFB in OH, the 911th TAG located at Pittsburgh International Airport in Pennsylvania, or the 731st Tactical Airlift Squadron (TAS) at Westover AFB in Massachusetts. The C-123s transferred to TAGs or TASs were used between 1972 and 1982 by AF Reserve personnel for military airlifts, medical transport, and cargo transport in the United States and internationally. Thirteen former ORH C-123s were sold through the Military Assistance Program to other countries, including El Salvador, Korea, Laos, the Philippines, South Vietnam, and Thailand (detailed information is included in Table B-1 in Appendix B).

AF Reserve Work Practices on Repurposed C-123s

Between 1972 and 1982, approximately 1,500–2,100 AF Reservists worked aboard C-123 aircraft that had previously been used to spray herbicides in Vietnam. It has been estimated that approximately one-third of all the C-123 aircraft used by the AF Reservists were former ORH planes (Alvin L. Young, A.L. Young Consulting, Inc., personal communication, August 10, 2014). The AF Reserve crews were assigned to different aircraft for each mission so it is likely that they spent time in ORH C-123s sometime during their service (Carter, 2014b). The committee notes that even if the ORH C-123s constituted less than one-third of a unit's fleet, with random assignment of planes for each mission, the probability of never serving on an ORH C-123 after a dozen or so missions is 0.013. Traditional AF Reservists worked one weekend per month plus one 2-week training session annually. Some maintenance and flight crews worked 5–10 days per month and other maintenance and flight crews worked full-time, either as Reservists or as Air Reserve Technicians (Carter, 2014a). Each C-123 flight crew included a pilot, navigator, flight engineer, and a loadmaster. In addition to the flight crew, maintenance personnel, paratroopers, and aero-medical personnel (including nurses), all had duties which could have brought them in contact with former ORH C-123s (Alvin L. Young, A.L. Young Consulting, Inc., personal communication, May 5, 2014).

The length of time the AF Reserve crew members spent aboard C-123s (both in flight and on the ground) could vary from 4.5 to 12 hours per shift depending on the mission or circumstances (Carter, 2014b). Typical pilot training and aeromedical evacuation missions were 4 hours in length; missions involving transport of weapons, explosives, or vehicles could be much longer. Cross country training missions were typically 4–7 hours to reach a specific destination away from home base. Deployments to Europe or South America lasting up to 12 hours in length were conducted with extended range fuel tanks (Carter, 2014b).

According to former AF Reservists, a flight mechanic would complete a 1.5-hour preflight inspection prior to each mission. Loadmasters required approximately 1.5 hours to prepare for aeromedical evacuations or missions involving an air drop of cargo or personnel. Static ground training missions held on the tarmac required crews to remain in C-123s for long periods of time. These immobile training sessions, during which crew members would rotate through different crew positions for training purposes, could last as long as a regular in-flight mission. For medical missions, aircrew would test medical systems, place litter straps and stanchions in place, and load, test, and store equipment. Medical personnel had contact with the floor while working along gurneys that were close to the floor. During training missions, the AF Reservists simulated patients who were loaded and "treated" in flight. During routine flight operations, flight crews sat on the floor, reclined, kneeled, sat on bucket seats, or crawled while completing their duties or doing maintenance work. Crew members routinely touched the deck, top, and sides of the aircraft interior. Maintenance personnel were even more intensely in contact with the aircraft interior surfaces (Carter, 2014a). Maintenance workers were tasked with painting, sheet metal work, wiring, grinding, fabricating, component replacement, complex welding, fabric work, anti-corrosion, alignment, and tuning.

C-123 crew members were issued Nomex™ flight suits, jackets, and gloves that were similar to those worn by other airplane crews. The Nomex™ flame resistant flight suits were not designed to protect the flight crews from chemical exposures; gloves could be removed and sleeves could be rolled up. After flight, the suits were handled, laundered, and stored by the individual crew members. Because C-123 aircraft were neither heated nor air-conditioned, winter operations typically required long johns, parkas or winter flight jackets, wool watch caps, and winter flying boots. No hazmat gear was issued, but maintenance personnel would wear appropriate protection for specific ground tasks (for example painting, cleaning or filling fuel tanks, or working with anti-corrosives).

Reservists typically brought their meals with them on flights, which were stored in the cooler tail sections of the aircraft because no refrigeration facilities were on board. Meals, which were usually sandwiches, were consumed while in flight. Fresh coffee and water were provided for each flight. There were no sanitation facilities inside the aircraft and only moist towlettes were available for personal hygiene.

The committee notes that **a considerable amount of information necessary for meaningful quantitative estimation of the Reservists' exposure proved not to be recoverable at all or remained resistant to reconciliation** of the content provided by various sources. For instance, considerable effort by a number of parties has failed to establish exactly how many C-123s the military had in Vietnam; how many were used for spraying herbicides (the ones referred to in this report as ORH C-123s); how many sprayed only insecticides; how many were returned to the United States; how many ORH C-123s and how many C-123s that had not been in Vietnam were allocated to the various reserve units.

CONCERNS ARISE ABOUT EXPOSURE TO HERBICIDES

Air Force Health Study

In 1979, a commitment was made by the AF to study potential adverse health effects in ORH personnel (AFHS, 1982). No exposure information was available for this cohort; no air or wipe samples were taken from ORH aircraft while being used in Vietnam. After an extended peer review process, the Air Force Health Study (AFHS) protocol was approved in 1982 calling for a matched-cohort design in a nonconcurrent prospective setting to evaluate morbidity, mortality, and reproductive health in ORH veterans (AFHS, 1982). The AFHS protocol called for six comprehensive physical examinations to be completed within a 20-year period.

According to an AF Working Paper prepared by the USAF School of Aerospace Medicine, the AF Reserve population was initially considered as a comparison population for the AFHS, but was dropped from consideration because the population was too small (identified as less than 3,000 people) and because "many of the Ranch Hand aircraft were reconfigured for transport and insecticide missions and thus, non-Ranch Hand crews responsible for these other missions, may have been exposed to significant Herbicide Orange residues in these aircraft . . . this group may not have been truly unexposed to herbicides, and was discarded as an appropriate control population" (AF Working Paper, 1979, p. V-4). AF personnel who flew C-130 aircraft in Southeast Asia during the same time as ORH personnel were eventually selected as the comparison population for the AFHS.

The initial study population consisted of 1,269 ORHs and 24,971 comparison veterans, nonexposed AF veterans who served in Southeast Asia between 1962 and 1971 (AFHS, 1983). During the course of the six examination cycles—in 1979, 1982, 1987, 1992, 1997, and 2002—more than 80,000 biological specimens were collected and stored and 1,800 serum TCDD concentrations were measured in ORH veterans who had blood draws (AFHS, 1991, 1995, 2000; Robinson et al., 2006).

Although several epidemiologic studies were published on AFHS physical examination results, few significant findings have been reported in ORH veterans. Diabetes, described as "the most important dioxin-related health problem seen in the AFHS," was found to be 21% higher in AFHS participants when compared to the comparison group (AFHS, 2005; Michalek and Pavuk, 2008). The various epidemiological studies of the ORH cohort generally lack the power to detect elevated cancer rates consistent with doses reconstructed from biomonitoring and the carcinogenic slope factor last endorsed by US Environmental Protection Agency (EPA, 2012). Therefore, **lack of positive epidemiological evidence in ORH personnel** (itself a matter of some dispute) **does not preclude an elevated carcinogenic risk for the AF Reservists,** particularly because TCDD has been found to be carcinogenic to humans by the International Agency for Research on Cancer (McGregor et al., 1998) and no safe level has been determined.

The experience of ORH personnel, both during their service in Vietnam and as participants in the AFHS, provides important historical context for how C-123 aircraft became contaminated with herbicides and how the unique exposure of the ORH cohort may have impacted their health. It must be noted, however, that the experience of ORH personnel is peripheral to the current committee's charge. This Institute of Medicine (IOM) committee is charged with examining the potential exposure of AF Reserve personnel who worked and trained aboard C-123 aircraft that were used by ORH personnel for herbicide spray operations in Vietnam. The determination of any potential exposure—or level of exposure—of AF Reserve personnel were considered by an evaluation of data that is directly relevant to their unique exposure opportunity. Their daily work environment was aboard C-123 aircraft that were formerly used to spray herbicides and samples taken of these aircraft indicate that chemical residues remained. The potential exposures for AF Reserve personnel were evaluated strictly on that basis by this committee, not by direct extrapolation from the health experience of ORH personnel.

RESIDUAL CHEMICALS IN FORMER ORH AIRCRAFT

Existing Sampling Data

"Patches" Sampling Data (1975, 1979)

Among the C-123s used by AF Reserve personnel between 1972 and 1982, was "Patches" (aircraft tail number 56-4362). "Patches" was hit more than 500 times by enemy ground fire while being flown for ORH defoliation missions in Vietnam, and earned its nickname for the numerous metal patches applied to cover and repair its many holes (Cecil and Young, 2008). Most flight records and historical documents provided to the committee indicated that "Patches" flew herbicides missions in Vietnam from 1961–1965 (USAF, 1979; Young and Young, 2014a); although at least one record reproduced from the USAF Historical Records Research Agency indicated that "Patches" was not converted to spray herbicides or insecticides until 1967 (Carter, 2013). After 1967, "Patches" was assigned to insecticide spray missions in South Vietnam as part of Operation FLYSWATTER (Young and Young, 2014a).

Several AF Reserve personnel recall flying on former ORH C-123s that had an "overwhelming chemical smell," and "Patches" was one of the C-123s reported to have objectionable chemical smells in its cabin (Battista, 2014; Carter 2013; Cecil and Young, 2008). Although TCDD is odorless and colorless, Cecil and Young (2008) described "Patches" as "reeking of malathion" that remained after years of spraying the insecticide while flying in Vietnam as part of Operation FLYSWATTER. Accounts from AF Reserve personnel, however, identified the odor as being from AO residue remaining in the aircraft (Battista, 2014; Carter, 2013).

In 1975, a "black, viscous, odorous residue" was found in "Patches" while it was undergoing a depot level wing modification at Hayes International Corporation in Dothan, Alabama. A sample of the residue, analyzed by the USAF Environmental Health Laboratory at Kelly AFB, was determined to be malathion; no "Herbicide Orange" was identified in the sample (USAF, 1979). Detailed results from this analysis were not made available to the committee.

In April 1979, after crews from the 439th Tactical Air Command Hospital complained about chemical odors while flying in "Patches," air and scrape samples were collected and evaluated for Herbicide Orange (specifically testing for 2,4,5-T and 2,4-D) and malathion (USAF, 1979). Surface loadings and air concentrations determined that 2,4,5-T butyl ester and 2,4-D isooctyl ester were present at sub mg/m^3 quantities in the air and in paint scrapings (90 to 150 μg/kg) from cargo tie-down rings, documenting that these phenoxy herbicides were still present in the aircraft (see Table 3-2). The phenoxy herbicides 2,4-D butyl ester and 2,4-D isooctyl ester were components of AO and AO II, respectively, which were sprayed in Vietnam by ORH. Based on the records of sampling, these three air samples were collected over a 5-hour period while the aircraft was stationary. The air samples were collected using chromosorb (c1-2), which collects the vapor phase and (because no filter was specified in front of the tube) particulate matter. TCDD was not analyzed in the air or in paint scraping samples in 1979 (because sufficiently sensitive analytic methods for identifying dioxin would not be developed until the 1980s, and even then the cost to analyze each sample was on the order of $1,000). The AF reported that the test results were low enough to "indicate no health hazard."

TABLE 3-2 Interior Sampling for Phenoxy Herbicides of C-123 Planes Used in Operation Ranch Hand

Source	C-123 Tail Number	2,4,5-T	2,4-D	Location
		Herbicide Air Samples (mg/m^3)[a]		
USAF (1979)	56-4362[a,b]	0.14	0.11	Front starboard, 3 ft. above floor
		0.19	0.23	Middle port, 3 ft. above floor
		ND	ND	Rear starboard, 3 ft. above floor
USAF (2009b)	55-4532	ND[c]	ND[c]	Interior
	55-4571	ND[c]	ND[c]	Interior
		Herbicide Scrape Samples (μg/kg)		
USAF (1979)	56-4362[b]	~ 150[d]	~ 92[e]	Cargo tiedown ring, center of plane
		< 60[f]	< 60[e]	Cargo tiedown ring, center of plane
		Herbicide Wipe Samples (μg/m^2)		
USAF (1996)	54-0607	2,600	3,400	Spray line, right
		< 95	< 81	Floor, right
	54-0618	130	< 81	Sprayline, left
		< 95	< 81	Floor, right
	54-0586	1,400	8,600	Spray line, right
		280	430	Floor, right
	54-0628	< 95	< 81	Sprayline, left
		< 95	< 81	Floor, right

TABLE 3-2 Continued

Source	C-123 Tail Number	2,4,5-T	2,4-D	Location
	54-0693	—	—	Spray line, right
		2,600	3,100	Floor, left
	54-0701	1,000	7,700	Spray line, right
		< 95	100	Floor, right
	55-4520	290	240	Spray line, left
		1,400	2,200	Floor, left
	55-4532	560	1,100	Spray line, right
		430	650	Floor, right
	55-4571	< 95	130	Spray line, right
		650	600	Floor, right
	55-4577	41,000	38,000	Spray line, right
		220	140	Floor, right
	56-4371	1,500	< 900	Sprayline, right
		220	< 81	Floor, left
	55-4547	< 95	< 81	Spray line, right
		< 95	< 81	Floor, right
USAF (2009b)	55-4532	1,000	810	Interior floor-1
		100	< 500	Interior floor-2
		240	140	Interior floor-3
		1,100	1,200	Interior floor-4
		650	560	Front bulkhead wall
		37	< 500	Interior ceiling (between wings)
		390	450	Interior rear frame
	55-4571	490	540	Interior floor-1
		100	110	Interior floor-2
		360	520	Interior floor-3
		310	250	Interior floor-4
		260	180	Front bulkhead wall
		600	1,600	Interior ceiling (between wings)
		720	100	Interior rear frame-1
		840	780	Interior rear frame-2
		980	1,200	Interior rear frame-3

[a] The air sampling methods used on these two occasions differed, so results are not fully comparable.
[b] C-123, Tail Number 56-4362 is known as "Patches."
[c] Detection limit not provided.
[d] Detection limit provided but in incorrect units. Stated as 1 μg/100 m^2 for 2,4,5-T and 4 μg/100 m^2 for 2,4-D.
[e] Butyl ester.
[f] Isooctyl ester.

"Patches" Sampling Data (1994, 1995)

In 1980, the Air Force moved "Patches" to museum status and transferred the aircraft to the USAF Museum (renamed the National Museum of the USAF in 2004) located at the Wright-Patterson AFB in Dayton, Ohio, where it was displayed outside because of residual chemical odors (Cecil and Young, 2008). Additional sampling of "Patches" was undertaken in 1994 when plans were under way for repair work to the aircraft and it was slated to be moved to an indoor display at the museum. For the protection of aircraft restoration personnel, wipe samples were taken from the interior and exterior of the aircraft prior to starting restoration efforts. There was some indication that the sample collection sites were in the section of the aircraft where AO is likely to have been spilled or leaked during spray operations (USAF, 1994). Sampling locations were from "areas of limited traffic near the agent orange spraying equipment" and these areas were "somewhat protective of routine crew movement and routine historical maintenance" (USAF, 1994). The 1994 sampling found TCDD in the interior of the aircraft, but not on the exterior. The absence of TCDD on the exterior is consistent with its photo-degrading in sunlight. The three interior TCDD measurements spanned a wide range (200 to 1,400 ng/m^2) (see Table 3-3), and were determined to likely "be representative of other locations of limited traffic near the agent orange spraying equipment," but not considered to be "indicative of the surface contamination throughout the entire cargo area of the aircraft" (USAF, 1994). As a result of the 1994 sampling, "Patches" was determined to be "highly contaminated" with polychlorinated dibenzodioxins (USAF, 1994). Restoration work was recommended for decontamination of the aircraft using protective equipment and processes for containment of contaminated dust. Thereafter, public entry was prohibited (USAF, 1994).

In a letter to the editor by Nieman (2014) concerning an article about potential exposures aboard former ORH C-123s by Lurker et al. (2014), it was revealed that there had been additional sampling of "Patches" in 1995; information about this episode of sampling and the results (USAF, 1995a,b,c) were provided to the committee on May 15, 2014. Samples collected in 1995 from "Patches" were analyzed as composite samples of between three and six wipe samples. Each group was collected from different sections of the aircraft, five from the interior sections and five from exterior sections. Four of the interior composite samples, collected from the front and mid-section of the aircraft were below detection limits (< 12 to < 20 ng/m^2). The fifth interior composite sample, collected from the rear of the aircraft, found a concentration of 30 ng/m^2. The 1995 sampling results are presented in Table 3-3.

The reason for the substantial differences in TCDD surface loadings measured in 1994 and 1995 in "Patches" are unclear. There could have been unidentified inconsistencies in sampling or analysis methods. No details on the collection protocols for the 1995 samples were provided. If a dry or water wipe was used

TABLE 3-3 Interior Sampling for TCDD of C-123 Planes Used in Operation Ranch Hand

Source	C-123 Tail Number	Concentration[a]	Location
		TCDD Air Samples (pg/m³)	
USAF (2009b)	55-4571	< 4.5	Interior
	55-4532	< 4.1	Interior
		TCDD Wipe Samples (ng)	
USAF (1996)	unknown	0.21[b]	Auxiliary power unit
		6.9[b]	Metal railing top of tank
		TCDD Wipe Samples (ng/m²)	
USAF (1994)	56-4362[c]	200	Horizontal surfaces "from areas
		250	somewhat protective of routine
		1,400	crew movement"
USAF (1995a,b,c)	56-4362[c]	30	Interior rear
		< 15	Front port
		< 12	Front starboard
		< 20	Center port
		< 13	Center starboard
USAF (2009b)	55-4532	24	Interior floor-1
		25	Interior floor-2
		28	Interior floor-3
		12	Interior floor-4
		4.8	Front bulkhead wall
		8.1	Interior ceiling (between wings)
		13	Interior rear frame
	55-4571	18	Interior floor-1
		27	Interior floor-2
		21	Interior floor-3
		4.3	Interior floor-4
		7.1	Front bulkhead wall
		1.0	Interior ceiling (between wings)
		9.3	Interior rear frame-1
		32	Interior rear frame-2
		10	Interior rear frame-3

[a] It might have been preferable to consider TCDD results in terms of Toxicity Equivalency Quotients (TEQs) from all dioxin, furan, and PCB congeners with "dioxin-like activity" through the aryl hydrocarbon receptor (AHR), as did Lurker et al. (2014). However, TEQs were not available from the 1995 and 1996 TCDD sampling events; results of the 1995 sampling were made known only after the publication of Lurker et al. (2014), and, for the reason explained in the next footnote, the 1996 sampling results were not suitable for use in calculating exposure.

[b] Collected samples were positive for TCDD, but area sampled was not reported so loading (mass/area) cannot be calculated.

[c] The C-123 with tail number 56-4362 is known as "Patches."

rather than a solvent (hexane) wetted wipe, then the results would be expected to be lower. The original contamination was not uniform throughout the interior of the aircraft. Any loss by degradation or cleaning also may not have functioned evenly over the surfaces, thus making the very limited number of samples susceptible to perturbation by "hot spots." As noted in Chapter 2, TCDD and herbicides are semi-volatile, and so can be redistributed within the aircraft from volatilization/deposition with heating and cooling of the aircraft left outside the sun. Unlike the two C-123s sampled in 2009, "Patches" had not spent an extended time sealed up on the desert, so it would not have experienced this phenomenon that would contribute to more uniform distribution of the contaminants throughout the interior. "Patches" was thoroughly washed and decontaminated after this sampling effort took place, after which "no dioxin contamination was detected" (USAF, 1997a).

Sampling of Planes at Davis-Monthan AFB, Arizona (1996)

Between 1981 and 1986, 18 C-123 aircraft were retired to MASDC at Davis-Monthan AFB in Arizona (now called the 309th Aerospace Maintenance and Regeneration Group [AMARG]) for storage or possible sale. Of the 18 C-123 aircraft at MASDC, 13 were documented as having been used for ORH. For the remaining five (tail numbers 54-583, 54-585, 54-635, 54-685, and 55-4544), the records for one indicate that it had been used for spraying herbicide in Southeast Asia but not as part of ORH, three had no records suggesting they had ever been in Southeast Asia, and one had no aircraft records available (USAF, 2009a). Table B-1 (in Appendix B) provides a record of all 40 ORH aircraft that have been identified.

In May 1996, two wipe samples were gathered from the top of the auxiliary power unit and from the metal railing on top of the tank from one or two planes (no specification of aircraft tail number specified) and subsequently analyzed for TCDD (USAF, 1996). The measurements reported were 210 pg and 6,900 pg, but because the size of the surface area sampled was not provided, the surface loading could not be calculated (see Table 3-3). Wipe samples for 2,4-D and 2,4,5-T analysis were also collected using moist Whatman (6″× 6″) glass fiber filters from 17 of the 18 aircraft, of which 12 were ORH C-123s. The samples were collected from the floors under the spray line caps to evaluate the area likely to have had the maximum original deposition. Herbicides were detected in all the ORH aircraft (0.13 to 41 mg/m^2) (see Table 3-2). The presence of AO constituents in the 12 ORH C-123s 22 years after returning from Vietnam clearly demonstrated the lingering contamination of AO constituents, presumably including TCDD.

ORH Planes Sampled at Davis-Monthan AFB, Arizona (2009), and Disposition of C-123 Aircraft

After more than 20 years in storage at MASDC, the decision was made by the AF to recycle and dispose of the former ORH C-123 aircraft. Prior to the recycling, the AF sampled the planes "in the event of future liability issues and to protect personnel that may be involved in the recycling process" (USAF, 2009c). Four of the 18 C-123s were sampled using air sampling methods and wipe sampling for phenoxys (USAF, 2009a). Of these, two did not have documentation of having been used in ORH (tail numbers 54-0585 and 55-4544). Samples were collected from 100 cm^2 areas with pads wetted with hexane. Multiple locations were sampled in each aircraft. After analyzing 16 individual wipe samples, detectable levels of TCDD (with range of loadings on the floors from 4.3 to 28 ng/m^2 [mean 20 ng/m^2]) were detected in the two C-123 aircraft known to have been used in ORH and also found positive for phenoxys in 1996. TCDD loadings on other surfaces (wall, ceiling, rear frame) ranged from 1.0 to 32 ng/m^2 (see Table 3-3), whereas the two C-123 aircraft that did not have detectable TCDD were later determined to have no record of having sprayed herbicides in Vietnam (USAF, 2009b). The two planes with known use in ORH had mostly detectable levels of phenoxy herbicides (see Table 3-2).

In April 2010, the 18 C-123 aircraft stored at Davis-Monthan AFB were smelted at an off-base contractor-operated smelting unit for conversion to aluminum ingots (Young and Young, 2014a). Of the ORH C-123s identified in historical documents, only three remain in the United States. Those aircraft are located at museums in Delaware, Georgia, and Ohio (details in Appendix B, Table B-1).

Overall, when specified, **the current documentation indicated valid collection methods and valid analytical protocols were followed.** For estimating the loading on the surfaces, the committee decided that only data collected from aircraft used in ORH should be included. While the sampling sites were not equally distributed across all aircraft or locations within the aircraft, the committee considered all data available, particularly in light of the limited amount of sampling conducted on C-123 aircraft used in ORH, with concern for health risks focused on TCDD.

RETROSPECTIVE ESTIMATION OF CONCENTRATIONS FROM THE FULL SET OF WIPE SAMPLES

The measurements of TCDD from various interior surface locations on "Patches" or the other C-123 planes were variable (see Table 3-3). TCDD concentrations in surface wipe samples collected in C-123s between 1994 and 2009 ranged from 1,440 ng/m^2 in 1994 down to 1 ng/m^2 in 2009. The range among the 1994 samples alone was almost an order of magnitude (200–1,440 ng/m^2) (see Figure 3-1). Regardless of the actual reconditioning process for former ORH

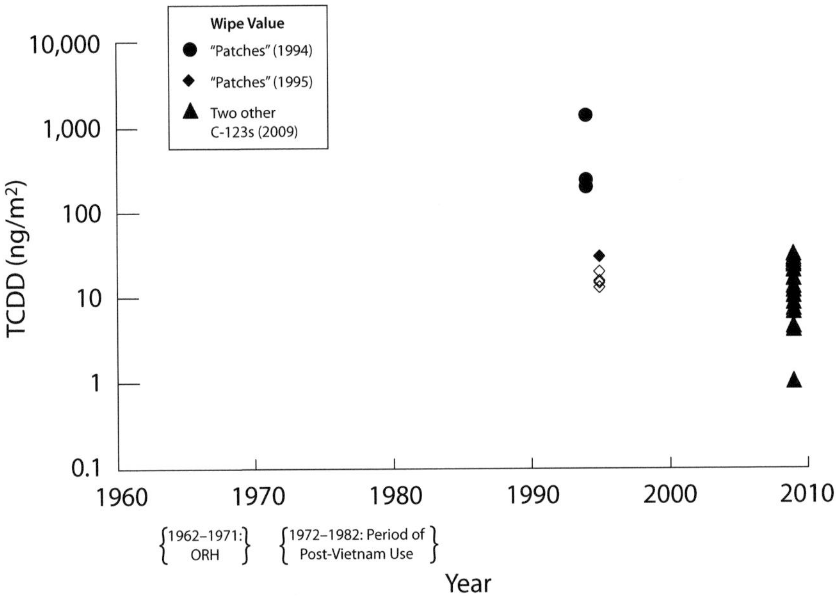

FIGURE 3-1 TCDD surface concentrations from interior wipe samples.
NOTE: TCDD surface concentrations obtained from the total of 24 wipe samples from the interiors of ORH C-123 aircraft by year. Clear points represent non-detect samples plotted at their detection limit.

C-123 aircraft, detection of TCDD in samples taken several decades later establish that any clean-up attempts had not been entirely successful. Records do not show that C-123 aircraft were tested for herbicide or dioxin contamination soon after they returned from Vietnam.

The committee noticed the singularly high TCDD value of 1,400 ng/m^2 reported in "Patches" in 1994. The samples collected in the same aircraft the following year had values considerably lower, with several below detection. These variations lead to uncertainty in estimating the actual exposures of the AF Reservists, but confirm that TCDD exposure would be expected. While some samples were collected in areas that are suggested to have had little traffic, the work patterns of the AF Reservists and the different configurations of equipment and personnel used in flight assignments led to the committee's judgment that contact with these surfaces carried a risk, though not quantifiable, of harmful exposure to the AF Reservists.

A number of limitations in these data are obvious. Samples were analyzed for TCDD only four times; 1994 and 1995 (from "Patches"), 1996, and 2009. The samples from "Patches" appear inconsistent, as far higher levels were found in

1994 compared to 1995 (the highest level measured in 1995 [30 ng/m^2] is more than 20-fold lower than the average level measured in 1994 [617 ng/m^2]). A major limitation is that the earliest TCDD samples were collected in 1994, roughly 20–25 years after these planes were returned from Vietnam and more than 10 years after their retirement from use by the AF Reservists in 1982. The committee agreed that the TCDD interior wipe samples were the most informative data available, although all of the TCDD samples from C-123s that were known to have been used in ORH came from a total of only three planes. Other aircraft known to have been used in ORH were not sampled for TCDD. The sampling sites within the planes were highly variable, and important details regarding collection and analysis methods were often found to be missing (see detailed discussion of samples above).

In addition to these TCDD wipe samples, air samples were collected in 2009 and analyzed for TCDD, all of which were non-detects, and samples from various media were collected and analyzed for 2,4-D and 2,4,5-T in 1979 and 2009 (see Table 3-2).

Clearly, any results of quantitative evaluation of potentially harmful TCDD exposures during the period of ORH C-123 use by the AF Reservists from such sparse and possibly inconsistent exposure data will be very uncertain. Therefore, the committee was unable to extrapolate with any confidence the levels of TCDD expected in the C-123s during 1972–1982 when exposure of the AF Reservists might have occurred.

Assuming there were no additional sources of TCDD contamination once the C-123s were returned to the United States, the discovery of residues long after ORH implies that degradation of TCDD was much slower within the planes than on their exteriors, which were exposed to sunlight and open environments. There is little doubt that TCDD surface levels in the late 1970s and early 1980s were higher than those in 1994, 1995, and 2009, and thus levels measured in these later years likely represent a lower bound on levels the AF Reservists might have been exposed to.

These factors led the committee to conclude the following:

Detection of TCDD long after the AF Reservists worked in the planes means that surface levels at the time of their exposure would have been at least as high as the available measurements, and quite plausibly considerably higher.

The resulting measurements of interior surface sampling in 1994, 1995, and 2009 most likely represent a lower bound, at least in terms of order of magnitude, of unit values of ng/m^2 for what the surface concentrations might have been when AF Reservists worked in the planes.

ASSESSMENT OF VALIDITY AND UTILITY

Wipe Samples

The ability of a wipe sample to capture true surface loadings is limited in many respects. It is likely that wipe sample data can differ, depending on the methods used in their collection (EPA, 1991) (i.e., different samplers, wiping material, solvent, or lab analyses), resulting in a wide range of values. In addition, there is variability due to specific characteristics of the sampled surfaces (e.g., porosity, texture, orientation) (CHPPM, 2009; EPA, 1991). The Environmental Protection Agency (1991) holds that even if adequate sampling is achieved, results are not always reproducible and estimates from wipe samples may indicate levels that are "substantially below true surface levels."

The utility of the wipe sampling of the C-123 aircraft is also reduced by the limited number of aircraft sampled and a limited number of surfaces sampled within each aircraft. For sampled surfaces, there is little information regarding the texture or porosity. Additionally, these samplings were conducted decades after the applicable time period of potential exposure. Sample collection methods were frequently either not reported (e.g., no mention of a wetting agent) or incompletely reported (e.g., solvent used is reported, but not the volume used), suggesting that methodologies across sampling periods were likely not uniform.

Air Samples

Air sampling methodologies vary depending upon whether the target compounds are expected to be present in the vapor or particle-bound phase. Particles are typically captured using filters that lack sorption capacity for vapor phase compounds. Vapor phase compounds are typically captured using a sorbent (porous polymer, polyurethane foam [PUF], etc.). Either type of sampler is encased in a cartridge with inlet and outlet ports through which air is drawn at a known rate. Sorbent cartridges will incidentally also capture particles, but are not considered reliable or quantitative for that purpose. When materials are expected to be present in both phases, use of a collection device consisting of a particle filter followed by a sorbent is standard practice.

Only very limited air sampling data were collected in the effort to understand potential post-Vietnam exposures in the C-123 aircraft. In 1979, air samples were collected from a single plane at Westover AFB in Massachusetts and analyzed for AO herbicides (and malathion). In 2009, particle samples were collected for herbicide analysis and vapor samples were collected for TCDD analysis from two ORH planes at Davis-Monthan AFB in Arizona.

The air sampling conducted in 1979 involved single air samples in three locations (sampled more or less simultaneously) within a single aircraft (tail number 56-4362) (USAF, 1979). The samplers utilized only a porous polymer sorbent (Chromosorb C-102). The samplers were operated for 5 hours at 0.74 liters per minute (lpm), producing sample volumes of approximately 0.2 m^3. The recorded temperature was 61°F and the elevation of Westover AFB is 243 feet above mean sea level. Two of the three samples revealed air concentrations of 2,4-D and 2,4,5-T that were near or above estimated vapor saturation concentrations of the acid moieties. However, the 2,4-D and 2,4,5-T esters have higher vapor pressures than the acids, and analysis of a scrape sample did reveal the presence of ester forms. Thus, the third sample was reported as non-detect, but a method quantitation limit was not reported. The third sample result is questionable. The samplers were all located within the open cargo area of the plane. Extreme concentration gradients are not plausible. The discrepancy is likely explained by sampling error (e.g., failure to collect or extract the non-detect sample) or an inadequate margin between the detection limit of the method and vapor saturation concentrations of the target compounds (i.e., poor sampling design). As noted above, measurable levels of 2,4-D and 2,4,5-T esters were found in a single surface sample collected by scraping, so despite the fact that no herbicides were detected in one of the air samples, a preponderance of the evidence suggests that herbicide was present in the air inside the plane during the 1979 sample collection.

In February 2009, additional air samples were collected from two other ORH C-123s (tail numbers 55-4532 and 55-4571) at Davis-Monthan AFB (USAF, 2009b). The temperature was not reported, but the average high and low temperatures in Tucson in February 2009 were 41°F and 75°F. The elevation of Davis-Monthan is approximately 2,700 feet above mean sea level. Herbicide samples were collected using Method 5001 of the National Institute for Occupational Safety and Health. This technique utilizes a glass fiber filter alone and does not capture vapor phase compounds. It is designed for capture of dusts of 2,4-D acid and 2,4,5-T acid. It does not capture the ester forms of the phenoxy herbicides. Samples were collected for 60 minutes at 2 lpm producing a sample volume of approximately 0.12 m^3. Results were reported as non-detect. Stated detection limits were roughly 8 and 30 $\mu g/m^3$ for 2,4,5-T and 2,4-D, respectively. Given that numbers in that range correspond to total suspended particulate concentrations encountered routinely in indoor environments such as homes and offices, and that sampling at Davis-Monthan was in planes not in active use (i.e., unoccupied), the sampling strategy may not have been sufficiently sensitive to detect herbicide unless the dusts captured approached 100% herbicide.

Air monitoring for TCDD on the two planes at Davis-Monthan in February 2009 followed EPA method TO-10a, which is a low volume PUF method for pesticides and PCBs. Sampling was conducted for 4 hours at 4 lpm, producing sample volumes of approximately 1 m^3. In contrast, the EPA method for PCDDs, TO-9a, specifies a sample volume of 325–400 m^3. Results were reported as non-detect for 2,3,7,8-TCDD in all four planes sampled. Detection limits of 0.5–4 pg/m^3 (0.0005–0.004 ng/m^3) were reported for TCDD. Documentation of quantitation limits was not provided and no positive (spiked) controls were reported. Therefore, evidence of extractability of TCDD from PUF using the applied methods was not provided. Per EPA method TO-10a guidance, detection limits of 0.001–50 μg/m^3 (1–50,000 ng/m^3) are expected with sampling times of 4–24 hours. Although limits are compound specific, the low end of that range is roughly 1,000 times higher than the detection limit claimed in the Davis-Monthan report.

These samples were collected to assess whether there was a significant exposure risk to personnel who were going to be involved in the destruction and recycling of the aircraft over a short period of time, rather than for exposures continuing over years, as was the situation for the AF Reservists. Also, given the low vapor pressure of TCDD, the unknown sampling temperature (vapor pressure declines with temperature), the high elevation of the site (lowered total pressure), lack of active personnel in the plane, and the extended period since service in Vietnam, the air sampling protocol was not appropriate to estimate inhalation exposure to the AF Reservists.

4

Evaluation of Assessments of Possible Exposure of Air Force Reservists from Service in Operation Ranch Hand C-123s

"The exposure assessment seeks to quantify the amount of a chemical contacting the outer boundary of a human and can provide an estimate of internal dose."

—TG 312 (CHPPM, 2009, p. 12)

Before the US Department of Veteran Affairs (VA) asked the Institute of Medicine (IOM) to convene this committee, a number of parties had expressed opinions about the sampling results[1] from C-123 aircraft that were formerly used to spray herbicides in Vietnam and were subsequently used by Air Force (AF) Reserve personnel in the United States between 1972 and 1982 (detailed sample results are presented in Chapter 3 of this report). The positions developed were based on qualitative, or at most semi-quantitative, treatment of the sampling data and their sources fall into two general categories:

- interpretations by individuals and entities associated with the military (USAF, 1994, 1997b, 2009a,b, 2012a,b; Young and Young, 2012, 2013a), and
- statements provided to the C-123 Veterans Association (ATSDR, 2012, 2013a,b; Berman, 2011; NIEHS, 2011, 2013; Schecter, 2013; Stellman, 2012, 2013).

[1] The one exception is that the results of a second dioxin sampling of "Patches" in 1995 were not entered into the data set until spring of 2014, when their existence was pointed out by Nieman (2014) in a letter to the editor responding to Lurker et al. (2014).

In this chapter, the committee reviews the approaches adopted in these documents.

Just as this committee started its work, Lurker et al. (2014) published a paper that used the available C-123 sampling data in a much more quantitative fashion in three models of exposure. The strengths and weakness of these estimation models are also addressed in this chapter.

The committee then compares the existing indoor contamination guidelines for 2,3,7,8-tetrachlorodibenzo-*p*-dioxin (TCDD) (as presented in Table 2-1) to the range of exposures supported by the existing sampling data. This serves to put in context the degree to which the AF Reservists may be at increased risk of adverse health consequences in association with exposure to components of the herbicides sprayed in Vietnam from working in Operation Ranch Hand (ORH) planes after they were returned to the United States.

This chapter concludes with the committee's integration of these various pieces of information in a qualitative fashion. From this, the committee makes its judgment about whether the existing information related to sampling of the ORH C-123s support there having been a meaningful elevation in the risk of adverse health effect among the AF Reservists.

INTERPRETATIONS OF SAMPLING RESULTS BY ENTITIES ASSOCIATED WITH THE MILITARY

Between 1979 and 2009, air and wipe samples were taken from several C-123 aircraft that had formerly been used to spray herbicides in Vietnam and were then used by the AF Reservists in the United States from 1972–1982. These sampling efforts are detailed in Chapter 3 of this report. Internal memos, evaluations, and laboratory reports provided by the VA regarding the sampling included some comments regarding elevated levels, but their bottom lines were largely dismissive about the possibility of there being potential health hazards related to exposures to these aircraft. Specific instances are noted below:

- After noting that the results for 2,4-D and 2,4,5-T in air were below the 10 mg/m^3 threshold limit value for each of these herbicides, the conclusion was "Sample results show contamination levels to be below amounts considered to be possible health hazards" (USAF, 1979).
- Another AF report concluded "the interior of the C-123 aircraft under discussion is heavily contaminated with PCDDs." When referring to the 25 ng/m^2 standard for office workers established by the National Research Council (NRC) (1988) as applied to 70-kg restoration workers for 375 days, however, the report also noted that "a higher surface concentration would be acceptable" and recommended that, during restoration, exposure "be maintained at the lowest possible level" by use of protective gear and procedures (USAF, 1994).

- "[T]he C-123 exterior and the majority of the interior are not contaminated with PCDDs or PCDFs above detectable levels . . . contamination is confined to a very small area of the plane's interior and to the inside of the rear inspection ports" (USAF, 1995a).
- A consultative letter (USAF, 1997b) addressing the 1996 sampling at Davis-Monthan Air Force Base (AFB) of two ORH C-123s for TCDD and 12 for phenoxy herbicides, concluded that "there is potential for individual exposure" and that, before sale or transfer, at least 10 TCDD samples should be gathered from each plane and any with detectable dioxin needed to be fully decontaminated.

Reports in Preparation for Smelting of C-123s at Monthan-Davis AFB

In 2009, air and surface sampling was conducted for TCDD and phenoxy herbicides in 2 ORH C-123s and another 10 ORH C-123s were tested only for herbicide residues on surfaces (USAF, 2009a,b). The final report concluded that "concentrations of 2,4-D and 2,4,5-T detected inside the aircraft were very low with respect to risk-based screening levels of concern and do not pose a significant risk" and that "low levels of dioxin/furans, near the risk-based screening level, on all interior surfaces that were sampled" represent "low level contamination that does not pose a significant risk to personnel involved in short term recycling activities" (USAF, 2009b). No comments were made about the experience of the AF Reservists.

The risk-based screening levels presented in the 2009 USAF report (USAF, 2009b, Appendix F, and reproduced here in Table 4-1) were said to incorporate consideration of both oral and dermal exposure resulting from contaminated surfaces. The committee has determined that the aggregate screening levels derived from the pathway-specific surface contamination screening levels for the dermal and oral routes shown in Table 4-1 were calculated incorrectly. The USAF report calculated the screening levels by simply adding the individual screening levels for the two routes, rather than by using the inverse-of-the-sum-of-the-inverses formula, which is the US Environmental Protection Agency's (EPA's) recommended method for calculating aggregate screening levels (EPA, 2001).

As a result, the screening levels used were established on the basis of the less sensitive rather than the more sensitive of the two pathways; hence the derived guideline levels are not necessarily protective. Had the aggregate screening levels been calculated correctly from the stated dermal and oral screening levels, the TCDD result would be 1 ng/m^2 and the results for 2,4-D and 2,4,5-T would be 200 μg/m^2. For the two C-123s sampled in 2009 (see Tables 3-2 and 3-3), the average surface contamination levels reported for TCDD (14 and 16 ng/m^2), 2,4-D (590 and 590 μg/m^2), and 2,4,5-T (520 and 500 μg/m^2) exceeded these values.

TABLE 4-1 AF Screening Levels the Assessment of Surface Contamination with Committee's Correction

Chemical	Dermal Screening Level	Oral Screening Level	Erroneous Aggregate Screening Level	Aggregate Screening Level Corrected by Committee	Averages for Two Sampled C-123s
2,4,5-Trichlorophenoxy acetic acid (2,4,5-T)	206 μg/m^2	100,000 μg/m^2 (100 mg/m^2)	100,000 μg/m^2 (100 mg/m^2)	200 μg/m^2	520 and 500 μg/m^2
2,4-Dichlorophenoxy acetic acid (2,4-D)	206 μg/m^2	100,000 μg/m^2 (100 mg/m^2)	100,000 μg/m^2 (100 mg/m^2)	200 μg/m^2	590 and 590 μg/m^2
Polychlorinated Dibenzodioxins	0.00111 μg/m^2 (1.11 ng/m^2)	0.022 μg/m^2 (22 ng/m^2)	0.0231 μg/m^2 (23 ng/m^2)	1 ng/m^2	15 and 16 ng/m^2

SOURCES: Appendix F: Risk Screening Level Assessment, Table 1 (USAF, 2009b,d).

US Air Force School of Aerospace Medicine Report

In April 2012, the US Air Force School of Aerospace Medicine released a report commissioned by the Headquarters Air Force Medical Support Agency detailing an exposure assessment related to Agent Orange (AO) for UC-123 aircraft previously used in support of ORH in Vietnam (USAF, 2012a). The cover memo to the report (USAF, 2012b) summarized that

- There was no relevant personal exposure or laboratory data found.
- [E]xisting information is inadequate to accurately determine individual exposure.
- [I]t is unlikely that the exposures experienced between 1972 and 1982 would have been sufficient to cause harm.
- Given the absence of a clear finding of potential harm, we believe it unnecessary to relay such individual findings to persons who had entered or worked on C-123s between 1972 and 1982, and who may be unaware of this assessment.

The USAF (2012a) review described the USAF sampling study conducted in 2009 as being the "most comprehensive" and it adopted the screening levels and the associated conclusions from the 2009 report as valid. The committee, however, has determined that these screening levels were incorrectly calculated (as described in the previous section) and therefore cannot be assumed as protective as asserted by the USAF review.

The USAF review (2012a) also concluded that the air sampling data for the phenoxy herbicides were "within acceptable exposure limits" although no air exposure limits were presented in this document, and it is not clear what exposure limits are being referred to by the authors. The committee has concluded that the air sampling data were minimal and of unknown quality. Two of three air samples from a former ORH C-123 were collected in 1979 and tested positive for herbicide exposure. In addition, air samples from two other ORH planes were collected in 2009, decades after the relevant period of exposure, using a low-volume screening protocol. Those samples were acquired at ambient temperature and pressure unlikely to be generally representative of in-flight work conditions of the AF Reservists. All the 2009 TCDD air samples (including blanks and controls) were reported as non-detect without corresponding quality assurance/quality control (QA/QC) materials, bringing into question whether the laboratory conducting the analysis could in fact capture and extract relevant amounts of TCDD with the sampling media used.

The Executive Summary of the USAF report concluded that, since there is a lack of TCDD "regulatory standard or consensus standard of practice . . . in the occupational health profession, application of wipe sampling data to estimate personal occupational exposures is not warranted" (USAF, 2012a, p. 4). The committee concurs that there is no agreed upon method for estimation of dose from wipe sampling data, but notes (as reviewed below) that multiple agencies and individuals have attempted to make such estimates. Based on those efforts, it is unreasonable in this case to assume that uncertainty regarding the threat presented by observed surface loads can be interpreted as evidence of negligible risk. Dismissal of the results from wipe sampling was not justified.

The last of the four points in the conclusions section of the report (USAF, 2012a, p. 5) reads:

> With the lack of epidemiological evidence and few sampling results related to HO contamination of the UC-123 aircraft between 1972 and 1982, our assessment of risk is dependent upon the findings of the National Academy of Sciences' Institute of Medicine RANCH HAND studies. It is reasonable to assume that any exposures associated with HO in post-Operation RANCH HAND utilization of the UC-123 would likely be less than exposures associated with HO during Operation RANCH HAND. Consistent with the findings of the National Academy of Sciences' Institute of Medicine biennial report (2010), it is reasonable to conclude that it is not possible to derive quantitative estimates of any increased health risks for those individuals who came into contact with the UC-123 aircraft from 1972 to 1982.

The committee finds this paragraph problematic in three respects:

- The report's "assessment of risk" could not have been "dependent upon the findings of the National Academy of Sciences' Institute of Medicine RANCH HAND studies" (USAF, 2012a); that work is officially known as the Air Force Health Study because it was conducted by the Air Force, and is in no way a product of the IOM or any other part of the National Academies.
- It asserts that "It is reasonable to assume that any exposures associated with HO [Herbicide Orange] in post-Operation RANCH HAND utilization of the UC-123 would likely be less than exposures associated with HO during Operation RANCH HAND" (USAF, 2012a). The committee agrees that workday exposures during active use of AO were likely greater than post-war exposures on a comparable task basis. However, ORH personnel were in Vietnam for a median of about 320 days (CDC, 1988), and undoubtedly did not access spray aircraft on every day of in-country service. Post-war exposures to AF Reservists would have been generally less frequent on an annual basis, but may have extended for up to 12 years. So some fraction of the AF Reservist cohort could have conceivably spent more time in contaminated C-123s than did some fraction of the ORH cohort (especially if the AF Reservists worked full-time or were scheduled for additional hours throughout the year). In addition, some post-war tasks

could have resulted in workday exposures that exceeded the workday exposures of some less-exposed ORH personnel (for example, flight crew officers) in terms of overall duration, more work inside the planes on the ground under conditions of reduced ventilation, etc.

- In asserting "Consistent with the findings of the National Academy of Sciences' Institute of Medicine biennial report ([Update] 2010), it is reasonable to conclude that it is not possible to derive quantitative estimates *of **any** increased health risks* [emphasis added] for" the AF Reserve personnel, the AF report (2012a) misrepresents the charge and determinations of the Veterans and Agent Orange (VAO) committee. The second task assigned to VAO committees by the 1991 Agent Orange Act was to estimate risk to Vietnam veterans for each specific adverse health outcome. These ***outcome-specific*** *risks* are what are being referred to in the statement "estimation of risks experienced by veterans exposed to the chemicals of interest during the Vietnam War is not feasible" (IOM, 2012, p. 11). Not only is determination of potency factors from epidemiologic results for each health problem far from being feasible, there are no exposure data to be drawn upon for non–Ranch Hand Vietnam veterans. In contrast, the issue concerning the AF Reservists and ORH C-123s is whether the risk of *adverse health outcomes of **any sort*** was elevated among those with potential exposure. This committee considers the sampling data for the AF Reserve C-123 population, albeit limited, to be an adequate basis for a qualitative exposure assessment and for some judgment about the overall health risk from TCDD exposure that the AF Reservists may have experienced, and so finds this justification for not doing so from the authors of the USAF report (2012a) to be invalid.

Investigations into the Allegations of Agent Orange/Dioxin Exposure from Former Ranch Hand Aircraft

In a report with the above title (Young and Young, 2012), a similarly named one on 2,4,5-T (Young and Young, 2013b), and a formal briefing document (Young and Young, 2013a), the VA's Compensation Service received an interpretation of the "dry" Agent Orange residues found on surfaces inside C-123s used by AF Reservists after their use in Vietnam, which has been incorporated onto VA's webpage concerning this issue (http://www.publichealth.va.gov/exposures/agentorange/locations/residue-c123-aircraft/scientific-review.asp; accessed August 21, 2015). The committee found this description of the chemical properties and behavior of TCDD and its propensity for dermal absorption to be inaccurate. Notable issues include the following:

- Young and Young often refer to TCDD residues as "dry" and immobile. Semi-volatile organic compounds (SVOCs) that are nominally solid at room temperature are generally not found in pure, crystalline form in the environment. Even below their melting point, dilute SVOCs do not crystallize and are found sorbed or dissolved in various matrices (Mackay, 2001). Because TCDD is not deliberately manufactured, but only exists as a very dilute contaminant, it would be expected to behave as a sub-cooled liquid rather than a solid. Therefore, it would not be immobile as Young and Young asserted.

- No attempts to investigate the removal efficiency of the selected method or of alternative methods for surface sampling for TCDD specifically have been reported. Unlike the irreversible binding of organics by activated carbon, binding to metals would be expected to be negligibly small. For instance, when investigating surface wiping techniques, Deziel et al. (2011) used stainless steel as a substrate to avoid issues associated with wiping porous surfaces, and Slayton et al. (1998) stated "wipe-sampling procedures provide semi-quantitative data for non-porous surfaces (i.e., metal) but are considered poor for porous surfaces (i.e., concrete)." The claim that hexane is required to remove TCDD from surfaces in the C-123s appears to be conjecture and not evidence-based.
- The assertion that "studies of dermal contact with TCDD have found that any exposures that occurred were 'negligible' because the skin is a major barrier to TCDD uptake, contributing less than 1% over the long term to the body burden" (Young and Young, 2012, p. 3) is based on interpretation of a Dow-funded study of the link between soil contamination and body burden in nonoccupationally exposed adults (Kimbrough et al., 2010). The passage conflates dermal exposure with exposure to contaminated soil. Kimbrough et al. do not discuss dermal absorption, dismissing it a priori as "a minor contributor to body burdens of the general population." However, dermal exposure can be an important source of exposure in occupational settings. For instance, the Dioxin Registry Report for the Dow manufacturing facility in Midland, Michigan (NIOSH, 1991) notes that "air sampling for chloracnegens were [sic] discontinued by 1966 because skin contact was recognized as the primary route of exposure." Similarly, Kerger et al. (1995) state "The available literature suggests that dermal uptake of dioxin in the workplace may be the primary source of occupational exposure." It should be further noted that, at least initially, the TCDD in the C-123s would have been dissolved in herbicides, which are themselves well-absorbed (Harris and Solomon, 1992; Moody et al., 1990) and that at no point would the surface matrix in the planes have been soil.
- The claim that TCDD is not volatile below its melting point is also incorrect. As discussed in Chapter 2, TCDD behaves like other SVOCs with similar physical-chemical properties. At room temperature, it is generally dissolved or sorbed into a film and is in constant flux around equilibrium with surrounding media.

STATEMENTS PROVIDED TO THE C-123 VETERANS ASSOCIATION

The C-123 Veterans Association (CVA) circulated the available sampling data to several dioxin researchers requesting replies regarding their interpretations of possible exposures (ATSDR, 2012, 2013a,b; Berman, 2011; NIEHS, 2011, 2013; Schecter, 2013; Stellman, 2012, 2013). The statements that were provided agreed with the CVA position that the sampling data support the possibility that the AF Reservists' risks of adverse health effects were increased by their service in ORH C-123s.

Interpretation of the Agency for Toxic Substances and Disease Registry

Prior to the publication of Lurker et al. (2014), which is discussed in the next section of this chapter, the most detailed response to the CVA came from the Agency for Toxic Substances and Disease Registry (ATSDR), which provided three documents with the same approach and conclusion (ATSDR, 2012, 2013a,b). The first from Sinks compared the average TCDD concentration from surface wipe samples collected from the interior of "Patches" (USAF, 1994) to TCDD screening guidelines corresponding to a 10^{-6} cancer risk, as recommended by the US Army Center for Health Promotion and Preventive Medicine (CHPPM) in Technical Guide 312 (TG 312) (CHPPM, 2009). TG 312 derived surface wipe screening levels (SWSLs) for 70-kg office workers over a 10-year period assuming exposure to contaminated surfaces through dermal contact and absorption, incidental ingestion by hand-to-mouth behaviors, and inhalation through breathing resuspended particulates. Environmental samples with concentrations above the SWSL for TCDD indicate the need for a more thorough health risk assessment.

ATSDR calculated an average TCDD surface concentration of 636 ng/m^2 for the three C-123 interior wipes collected in 1994. ATSDR concluded that this value exceeded the TG 312 screening guideline of 3.5 ng/m^2 by a factor of 182, which corresponds to a 200-fold greater cancer risk than the screening value. The opinions expressed in the initial report were subsequently upheld twice, first by Ikeda and by Portier (ATSDR 2013a,b), and again in a presentation to this committee on June 16, 2014, by Sinks (ATSDR, 2014).

The initial ATSDR opinion letter acknowledged the limitations of the available data, most notably the questionable representativeness of TCDD surface concentrations from the sampled C-123s to surface levels in the other ORH C-123s and the 20- to 40-year lag time between when the AF Reservists worked on them and collection of the comparison surface wipe samples. ATSDR further acknowledged a lack of information on flight crew activities, work histories and duration of work in C-123 aircraft, and minimal information regarding their interior environment at the time when the C-123s were used by the AF Reservists. Additionally, ATSDR noted that the TG 312 SWSL was derived from an office worker scenario, and thus, was likely to be under-protective for the TCDD exposures of the AF Reservist personnel when they worked inside the confined space of an aircraft. Representative exposure levels of the AF Reservists would depend on skin surface area, duration of exposure, hand washing, and food intake. In their June 2014 presentation to the committee, ATSDR additionally pointed out that the newly available sampling data had been collected from wipe samples from different aircraft and sequential sampling of the same surfaces in a given aircraft had not been conducted. Thus, it is not possible to infer degradation rates for TCDD on the sampled surfaces. Further, the purpose of the additional surface wipe sampling was for estimating exposure risk for personnel preparing the aircraft for destruction or recycling, not for retrospective evaluation of exposures to C-123 Reservists.

ATSDR's summary interpretation of the available information was as follows:

- inhalation exposures to TCDD in C-123 aircraft could not be excluded;
- aircrew operating in "this and similar environments were exposed to TCDD";
- it was not possible to accurately establish the degree of exposure (high or low), or the risk of adverse effects among C-123 AF Reserve flight crew;
- the contamination levels in 1994 in at least one plane greatly exceeded current Department of Defense screening guidelines; and
- the observed levels would likely have required the use of personal protective equipment or the grounding of these aircraft.

These observations from ATSDR are largely in accord with the committee's assessment of the available data. A comprehensive comparison of the wipe samples reviewed by ATSDR to the TG 312 screening guidelines is provided in Table 4-2.

CRITIQUES OF THREE MODELS PRESENTED IN LURKER ET AL. (2014)

The CVA had provided Jeanne Stellman with the then available data from sampling of the C-123s (that is, without the sampling conducted on "Patches" in 1995). Dr. Stellman and colleagues, Fred Berman and Richard Clapp, entered into collaboration with Peter Lurker, who had been involved in the sampling conducted on the C-123 aircraft at Monthan-Davis AFB. A report of this group's efforts to perform quantitative exposure estimation using these data (Lurker et al., 2014) was published just before this committee was convened.

Lurker et al. (2014) presented three modeling approaches to address potential exposures to C-123 flight crews and maintenance personnel in post-Vietnam operations. The first approach involves estimation of exposure due to hand-to-mouth contact using a protocol based generally on prior exposure assessment guidance from EPA (1989) developed for management of hazardous waste sites and more specifically on May et al. (2002) and US Army guidance in TG 312 (CHPPM,

TABLE 4-2 ATSDR's Comparison of Interior Surface Wipe Samples Collected from C-123 to Screening Guideline of 3.5 ng/m^2 TCDD from TG 312 (CHPPM, 2009)

	Location of Planes		
	Wright-Patterson AFB (USAF, 1994)	Davis-Monthan AFB (USAF, 1996)[a]	Davis-Monthan AFB (USAF, 2009b)
Number of Planes Sampled	1	2	2
Number of Samples Available	3	2	16
Observed Mean (ng/m^2)	640	380	16
Observed Range[b] (ng/m^2)	(210–1,440)	(20–740)	(1 to 28)
Observed-to-Screening Ratio	180	10.8	4.6

[a] This committee found these two sample readings without specification of the area sampled could not be compared with other results in units of ng/m^2.
[b] The range of surface wipe concentrations from each sampling period has been added by the committee.
SOURCES: ATSDR, 2012, 2013a,b, 2014.

2009) developed for evaluation of risks to office workers from exposure to chemicals on indoor work surfaces. The committee calls this the "Dermal-oral Direct Contact Model." Lurker et al.'s (2014) second approach evaluated the potential degree of vapor supersaturation of herbicides in air samples collected in a C-123 in 1979 and then predicted potential inhalation exposures to vapor and particle-bound TCDD. The committee calls this the "Maximum Saturation Vapor Pressure Model." Lurker et al.'s (2014) third model adapted the methodology of Little et al. (2012), which uses an approach based on thermodynamic arguments to predict indoor air concentrations from surface residues of SVOCs. The committee calls this the "Thermodynamic Emissions Model." Exposures that were predicted using this third model were again attributable solely to inhalation. Lurker et al. (2014) interpreted the results of their modeling as supporting the premise that the AF Reservists had experienced exposure to residual herbicide components that could have exceeded guidelines of EPA, The Netherlands, and the World Health Organization.

The committee endeavored to reproduce the estimates Lurker et al. reported from these three models as a means of validating the models and of gaining full understanding of the assumptions that were made. With the validated models, the committee was able to explore the sensitivity of their results to various scenarios and changes in assumptions. The committee found none of the estimation models assessed to be without weakness and considered no particular exposure scenarios for the AF Reservists to be well documented. Consequently, the committee members did not find any specific quantitative estimates likely to be representative of the range of exposures experienced and so refrained from presenting any quantitative exposure estimates that might be construed as representing predictions it favored for the AF Reservists' actual exposures. This decision is also in accord with the committee's charge to conduct a qualitative assessment.

Dermal-oral Direct Contact Model

Although abbreviated as "dioxin dermal-oral exposure," the first model in Lurker et al. (2014) can more appropriately be described as a dose estimate of non-dietary oral ingestion due to hand-to-mouth contacts. The model has roots in EPA's guidelines for risk assessments at Superfund sites (EPA, 1989). EPA's original equation for intake (*I*) in mg/kg body weight-day is

$$1 = C \times \frac{CR \times EFD}{BW} \times \frac{1}{AT} \tag{1}$$

where *CR* is the contact rate, *EFD* is exposure frequency and duration, *C* is the contaminant concentration, *BW* is body weight, and *AT*, the averaging time.

Lurker et al. (2014) added terms to correct for the sampling efficiency of the wipe technique for surface concentration estimation (FT_{we}), and to convert units representing surface area (CF_a) and expanded the terms for contact rate and for exposure frequency and duration in the original equation as follows:

- $CR = (SA)(FT_{ss})(FT_{sm})(FT_{re})(CF_{wt})(FT_{ga})$

  Here, *SA* is the exposed skin surface area, FT_{ss} is the fraction of the mass of the contaminant that is transferred from the surface to the skin, FT_{sm} is the fraction of skin area that touches the mouth, FT_{re} is the fraction of contaminant transferred from the skin to the mouth, CF_{wt} is a conversion factor, and FT_{ga} is the fraction of contaminant absorbed from the gastrointestinal tract.

- $EFD = (RH)(EF)(WD)(ED)$

  Terms used include *RH*, the probability of being on a Ranch Hand aircraft; *EF*, the count of hand-to-mouth events per day; *WD*, the number of work days per year; and *ED*, the duration of exposure.

The equation in Lurker et al. (2014)[2] after these substitutions is

$$1=\frac{(RH)(C_s)(CF_a)(SA)(FT_{ss})(FT_{sm})(CF_{wt})(FT_{ga})(EF)(WD)(ED)(FT_{re})}{(FT_{WE})(BW)(AT)} \quad (2)$$

May et al. (2002) and TG 312 (CHPPM, 2009) were both mentioned in Lurker et al. (2014) as sources that also had adapted EPA's intake model. The committee found that the three versions differ slightly in how they compute the ingestion due to hand-to-mouth events. Most notable are terms explicitly accounting for the frequency of contacts between the skin and surfaces (in the May model) and the fractional surface area involved in the contact between skin and surfaces (in the CHPPM model). Lurker's model does not seem to account for either of these factors. Aside from some confusion on the interpretation of this transfer input, the Lurker et al. (2014) model is specifically for non-dietary ingestion dose due to hand-to-mouth contacts. The model does not aim to include non-dietary ingestion due to object-to-mouth contacts, let alone inhalation, dermal, or dietary ingestion exposure. This exclusivity could be a problem when the contaminant of interest is assumed to reside in multiple media and where other routes of exposure may be important.

Additionally, this model embodies a simple linear estimate. The direction in which an increase or decrease in the value of any input variable will modify the resulting exposure estimate is entirely predictable. The model does not account for chemical-dependent properties (for example, transport, decay, partitioning) or uncertainty in input parameters. It can be used for individuals of different body weight, but aside from this, there are some restrictions in the ability to include varying activities (such as contact with surfaces) from person to person or over time.

This model is quite representative of commonly used models for exposure estimation, but almost any result could be obtained depending on what values are assumed for the large number of input variables. A broad spectrum of values is usually feasible for any exposure situation under investigation, but the extensive uncertainties about the actual work histories of the AF Reservists in this case make this model even more flexible. The committee agrees with the point made by Driver (Driver and Solomon, 2014) at the committee's workshop that with its multiplicity of component variables, each of which can be assigned a wide range of values, the model is too plastic to provide any real insight into what levels of exposure might actually have occurred.

---

[2] Personal communication with the authors confirmed that the term FT_{sm} was missing from Equation 2.

Maximum Saturation Vapor Pressure Model

The saturation vapor pressure model presented in Lurker et al. (2014) is a simple thermodynamic model premised on the assumption that the maximum vapor air concentration in an enclosed environment will be a function of the saturated vapor pressure. However, applying it to semi-volatile compounds in a mixture can present a number of challenges. In addition, the saturated vapor pressure is temperature- and pressure-dependent. To apply to an air concentration, a closed system is assumed with no air exchange. This is not the case when an aircraft is in use, however, so this pathway would represent a maximum concentration that would result through volatilization under static conditions. The herbicide 2,4-D or 2,4,5-T concentrations in the Lurker paper were derived by assuming each was a pure substance at 760 mm Hg air pressure. These substances are solids at room temperature. If they are dissolved in an oil-based film then the mole fraction of other compounds in the film with similar vapor pressure should be considered. Driver and Solomon (2014) noted that the air concentrations to which the calculated vapor pressures were being compared were not the acid forms of 2,4-D and 2,4,5-T, but rather the esters which have a considerably higher vapor pressure.

Based on the premise that the 2,4-D and 2,4,5-T acid vapor concentration calculated was lower than the measured concentration, the measured air concentration would contain both vapor phase and particulate phase of these compounds. The next step was to estimate the TCDD air concentration by assuming that, because the 2,4-D and 2,4,5-T were in both the vapor and particulate phase and TCDD is less volatile than either of the herbicides, it also would be partitioned from the vapor phase to a particulate phase. The committee was unable to reproduce the TCDD air concentrations reported in the Lurker paper by following the indicated calculations with the specified inputs. There are a number of questionable assumptions involved in these calculations. Driver and Solomon (2014) objected that the value used in the Lurker paper for the concentration of TCDD in AO represents the upper range of what has been found to have been present in AO. Lurker et al. (2014) also assumed that the degradation of TCDD within the aircraft was similar to that of the herbicides within the aircraft, which is questionable.

Independent of whether the model predicts appropriate saturated vapor pressure for TCDD, the applicability of this model for an inhalation route is questionable because, once the doors and hatch of the aircraft were opened, the air exchange would increase within the aircraft and while the aircraft was flying the increased air exchange would drastically reduce the air concentration associated with volatilization. The basic premise is that there would be redistribution onto particles of SVOCs with resulting exposure. However, the TCDD concentration on the particles cannot be determined by this method. The committee found that this model is unsuitable for estimation of exposures experienced while a contaminated plane was in flight and that its use is further hindered by the difficulty of establishing appropriate values for the saturation vapor pressure.

Thermodynamic Emissions Model

The third model in Lurker et al. (2014) was a general thermodynamic model developed for emission of SVOCs, a class of compounds that includes TCDD. The model is based on a screening level model described in Little et al. (2012), which was proposed for use in health-based evaluations of chemicals prior to entry into commerce. Lurker et al. (2014) applied this model by using an expected gas phase concentration immediately above the surface of the source material, the exchange between the air and organic film expected to be throughout the aircraft on surfaces and dust based on an octanol-water coefficient, the surface area of the interior of the aircraft, and the ventilation rate. This approach can provide a steady state air concentration in a specified microenvironment with a constant air exchange rate and a source of SVOCs that is not exhausted over the time period of interest.

This is an appropriate model to use for TCDD in the post-Vietnam ORH C-123 aircraft if the input parameters can be properly established. However, the committee identified problems for several of the input parameters presented in the Lurker paper:

- The value given in Table 6 of Lurker et al. (2014) for the convective mass-transfer coefficient (h) appears to be an order of magnitude low. Based on the air concentrations given in the paper, it appears that a value of 3.68 m/h (rather than the tabled value of 0.368 m/h) was actually used.
- The ventilation rate of 170 m^3/h, which is said to be adapted from Meek (1981), is much smaller than the ventilation rate of 8,464 m^3/h for a flying C-123 aircraft reported in that document. It should be noted that the crew were also in the aircraft before and after flights and during training session while on the ground when the ventilation rate would be only a fraction of the 170 m^3/h.
- The interior surface area was underestimated by assuming a cylindrical shape because portions of the interior were exposed substructure of the aircraft which present a much larger surface area than a smooth surface.
- The largest uncertainty is associated with y_0, the gas-phase concentration in contact with the emission surface, which was calculated using maximum saturation vapor.

As indicated above there are a number of problems with the assumptions in the Lurker paper calculations. Even if those values were accepted as accurate, Lurker et al. (2014) corrected the gas phase TCDD concentration for the portion that would be on the particle phase, which should not be included in y_0. Estimating y_0 is recognized as the largest shortcoming of this model approach (Little et al., 2012). Thus, the committee does not have confidence in the TCDD air concentrations calculated from this model based on the input parameters used.

The approach taken by Little et al. (2012) could, however, reasonably be applied to a scoping analysis of the inhalation exposures to the C-123 flight crews. Based on that approach, vapor phase air concentrations would be expected to be highest while planes were stationary and lowest during flight. Time spent in the planes while they were on the ground is, therefore, a key determinant of exposure due to inhalation and dermal absorption of vapor. Based on projected on-ground air concentrations, and given that aggregate exposures would be expected to be a multiple of vapor inhalation exposures, average workday exposures to flight crews could be problematic, but maintenance personnel whose on-ground time in the planes exceeded that of flight crews, or flight crews who participated in static training missions, probably had even higher exposures.

UNDERESTIMATES RESULTING FROM ALL POSSIBLE PATHWAYS NOT BEING FACTORED INTO SOME GUIDELINES

The committee used the existing indoor contamination guidelines for TCDD that were presented in Chapter 2 as a means of assessing the degree to which possible exposures of the AF Reservists may indicate possible adverse health consequences. The committee considered the guidelines for surface loading the most applicable to the occupational situation of the AF Reservists. These guidelines for surface loading range from 1 to 25 ng/m^2, with 3.5 ng/m^2 being the level derived by CHPPM and 22 ng/m^2 being the guideline derived in the 2009 AF report. (More correctly, the AF value should have been 1.1 ng/m^2, if dermal exposure actually had been taken into account; see Table 4-1.) Although such guidelines are derived with the intention of amply protecting the health of exposed individuals, some guidelines may not be as health-protective as the risk level nominally stated. The committee finds that the existing indoor contamination guidelines for TCDD (see Table 2-1) expressed in terms of surface loading or air levels are incomplete with respect to consideration of all possible exposure pathways.

Table 4-3 indicates which of all possible exposure pathways were factored into the guidelines derived for building re-entry, and which the committee found to be most applicable for the situation of the AF Reservists. Examination of the bases for the surface loading standards shows that they are largely driven by estimated ingestion exposures related to hand-to-mouth contact. Hand contamination is presumed to occur via contact with contaminated surfaces. Object-to-mouth contact is discussed in some of the relevant documents, but not actually included in dose estimation. Inhalation exposure is more often formally addressed, but typically not directly tied to surface contamination (even though, in a physical-chemical sense, air and surface residues are contiguous and exchanging phases). Hence, separate standards are derived for ingestion and inhalation pathways,

TABLE 4-3 Exposure Pathways Considered in Prior Surface Standard Relevant Literature

	Ingestion			Dermal Absorption	
	Hand-to-Mouth	Object-to-Mouth	Inhalation	Direct Contact	Vapor
Kim and Hawley (1985)[a]	√	—	√ [b]	√	—
CHPPM (2009)	√	—	√	√	—
WTC (2003)	√	—	√ [b]	√	—
Lurker et al. (2014)	√	—	√	—	—

[a] Adopted by NRC, 1988.
[b] Included but not explicitly linked to surface contamination.

with the proviso that measured contamination in either phase should lower the acceptable level of contamination in the other. Dermal exposure is often considered, but only as a consequence of direct contact with surfaces. As discussed below, dermal protocols use rates of contact with surfaces that are low compared to traditional values used in occupational and environmental health, assume that normal clothing is chemical-protective, and address dermal absorption in a crude manner. Dermal absorption of vapor-phase TCDD is not considered in any of the proposed protocols. Given that some potentially important pathways are ignored, and that others are treated in a perfunctory manner, the degree of protectiveness of the existing guidelines expressed in terms of surface loading or air concentration should not be assumed.

Transfer Coefficients

Transfer coefficients (TCs) are routinely used to characterize occupational exposure to contaminated surfaces. A TC represents the equivalent surface area from which 100% of the dislodgeable chemical residue is removed and transferred to the skin or clothing of a worker per unit of time. Application of this approach to assess the use of pesticides in indoor spaces is proceeding out of necessity, but is less firmly established than for agricultural applications due to greater heterogeneity in indoor surfaces and behavioral patterns. Nevertheless, methods for translating surface contamination to human dose are needed, and the TC approach is a likely candidate. Derivations of the guidelines for contamination of building interiors discussed here typically do not explicitly use an estimated TC (the 2003 World Trade Center [WTC] document is the exception). However, implicit transfer coefficients are inevitably found in all of the guidelines expressed in terms of surface loading. In agricultural occupational health practice, TCs routinely exceed 1,000 cm^2/hr. The WTC protocol utilized a TC of 1,200 cm^2/hr, but described it incorrectly as a skin contact rate and then inappropriately applied a surface-to-skin transfer efficiency.

Dermal Absorption of Residues on Skin

TCDD's rate of absorption into skin can be estimated from surface loads, transfer coefficients, and resulting predicted dermal doses. Fluxes are lower than available experimental results. For instance, the 3% availability assumed in the WTC protocol is based on absorption experiments conducted by Poiger and Schlatter (1980), who applied TCDD in soil to rats in vivo. Observed flux in the experiment producing the 3% estimate was nearly 500 pg/cm^2-hr or 10^6 times the flux implicit in the WTC protocol. Fraction absorbed is not independent of chemical load on skin (Kissel, 2011). Sampling skin surfaces with low loading is unlikely to provide an appropriate measure of potential dermal dose due to depletion, whereas testing at a high loading is unlikely to show dose dependence due to saturation. Application of fractional absorption data from high load experiments to low load conditions can lead to gross underestimation of absorption efficiency. Dermal absorption of the phenoxy herbicides has been shown to be substantial in laboratory animals and in human volunteers (Harris and Solomon, 1992; Moody et al., 1990); 2,4-D and 2,4,5-T penetrate the skin relatively rapidly and could potentially take TCDD with them. Dermal absorption of PCBs, which are chemically similar to TCDD, has been found to exceed bioaccessibilty via either the ingestion or respiratory route in humans (Ertl and Butte, 2012; Lees et al., 1987).

Dermal Absorption of Vapor

For compounds that are sparingly soluble in air, pulmonary absorption may or may not exceed absorption through the skin. Weschler and Nazaroff (2012) have presented methods for estimating the contribution of vapor absorption via skin to total exposure to vapor phase chemicals. Compounds for which absorption of vapor via skin might plausibly exceed absorption via inhalation include both TCDD and the n-butyl esters of the herbicides 2,4-D and 2,4,5-T.

PLAUSIBILITY OF AO-RELATED IMPAIRMENT OF HEALTH AMONG AF RESERVE PERSONNEL

With increasing awareness of the toxic potential of various agents in the environment, substantial resources have been expended to develop methods to evaluate health risks in a rational and consistent fashion. Over the past several decades a general framework has been accepted for developing quantitative guidelines (like those discussed in Chapter 2) for use in assessing exposures to toxic substances, but objectives vary and, by its very nature, risk assessment is fraught with uncertainties. Specific efforts in risk assessment invariably come to points of uncertainty where assumptions must be made and numerical inputs must be selected in order to move forward; however, opinions may differ on exactly what the appropriate decisions are in a given circumstance.

Given a range of options for addressing what could be concluded about health risks from the sparse set of results from exposure sampling on some of the C-123 aircraft that had been used in ORH and subsequently by AF Reservists, the committee undertook a number of approaches in an attempt to be inclusive and thorough. In the end, the committee reached the following consensus about the central question in this task: **It is plausible that working on these ORH C-123s could have contributed to adverse health effects for some AF Reservists.**

Historic reconstruction of occupational exposures relies on combining the two components of exposure, exposure concentration and contact time. Knowledge of the exposure levels during the time period of interest are combined with the job histories of the workers that delineate the time spent in the different activities (job classifications) that bring workers into contact with those exposure concentrations. Depending on the quality of the data available, the results can vary from a quantitative exposure evaluation usable for a quantitative risk assessment to a qualitative evaluation of whether a problematic exposure may have occurred. The data available to this committee fall into the latter category.

There were only limited numbers of measurements of TCDD and the herbicides in AO on the surfaces and in the air of aircraft flown by the AF Reservists (the exposure concentration), and those measurements were made years to decades after the exposures occurred. Although the paucity of measurements and delay in obtaining them increase the uncertainty about exposures, it is clear that decay and loss processes would result in overall lower levels at the time of measurement than had been the case when the AF Reservists actually were exposed. The committee, in the absence of knowledge of the losses of TCDD and herbicides during the time period of operation and storage of the aircraft, did not have a basis for predicting the decay in concentration and adjusting the measurements accordingly.

A second constraint on the committee's deliberations was an incomplete knowledge of which aircraft were employed by the AF Reservists, the specific jobs and activities they were involved in, and the duration of time spent in the aircraft during their service. These factors would have been needed to estimate the contact rate, frequency, and time. Thus, the committee based its conclusions on a qualitative evaluation of the AF Reservists' potential exposures, although quantitative estimates based on various models and assumptions were explored. **The committee considers the AF Reservists to have been exposed to TCDD and herbicide through multiple routes when on aircraft that had previously been used in ORH.**

A further consideration in interpreting the evidence is that background exposures were higher during the period that AF Reservists worked on the ORH

C-123s. In reaffirming its oral tolerable daily intake (TDI) of 2 pg/kg-d for TCDD and other dioxin-like chemicals, the Environment Agency of the United Kingdom (UKEA, 2009) noted that the average adult is estimated to consume about 49 pg TEQ from food and drinking water and to inhale approximately 0.2 pg TEQ on a daily basis, corresponding to a mean daily intake (MDI) of 0.7 pg/kg-d for a 70-kg adult. Twenty years earlier in 1988, the average person consumed on the order of 1.2 pg/kg-d TEQ (WHO estimate in NRC, 1988). Any AF Reservists ever assigned work on one of the ORH C-123s during their years of service most certainly received at least some increment in exposure to these substances. Superimposed upon the yet higher background levels of 1972–1982, such increments in exposure would have posed a more substantial threat to health than they would if experienced today. As discussed in Chapter 2, very small increments in exposure are not necessarily innocuous. They can increase the risk of adverse health effects either through a linear relationship or by crossing a threshold to a level at which adverse effects are plausible.

As another way of addressing its charge of putting in context the levels of exposure plausibly experienced by the AF Reservists, the committee attempted to compare them to existing guidelines for TCDD exposure within enclosed settings. When making such comparisons, the committee considered differences in the activities that influence exposures of the population for which the guidelines were developed, along with differences in duration of exposure. Such modulating activities include contact rates with surfaces, breathing rates, hand-to-mouth frequency, access to hygienic facilities before eating, surface area of the skin exposed, etc. Greater activity and movement of the AF Reservists would have resulted in contact with multiple surfaces since Reservists frequently sat on the floor of the aircraft with limited or no access to lavatory facilities prior to eating. This would suggest that they would have higher exposure from inadvertent ingestion and dermal pathways than office workers. On the other hand, the number of hours and years of work that the AF Reservists were in the aircraft were less that that used for establishing the guidelines for the office workers. Based on these varying conditions, it is the committee's judgment that it is plausible, in some cases, the AF Reservists' exposures exceeded TCDD guidelines for workers in enclosed settings.

All projected exposures will necessarily be uncertain due to limitations in the data available. The C-123 crews were potentially exposed to TCDD from air by inhalation and dermal absorption of vapors. Because of the methods used to collect the air samples, the committee did not consider the resulting measurements useful. Surface contamination with an SVOC can lead to exposure by inhalation of the chemical released into air, dermal absorption resulting from contacting a contaminated surface, and ingestion arising from hand-to-mouth transfer. There were 24 usable interior wipe samples of TCDD from ORH C-123s (see Table 3-3). Sixteen of them were collected in 2009, 27 years after the C-123s had been retired. The remaining eight were collected in 1994 and

1995, 12 years or more after retirement. These samples came from only three C-123s, and there is only a little anecdotal information on how representative these three C-123s are of all the ORH planes used back in the United States. There is no record of where in the interior of a C-123 some of the samples were collected. The three highest wipe samples (200, 250, and 1,400 ng/m^2 collected in 1994) seem rather inconsistent with five samples of the same plane conducted in 1995 for which the largest concentration measured was 30 ng/m^2, and the remaining four were non-detects (< 20 ng/m^2). Moreover, these samples were from "Patches," a plane selected for sampling because of chemical odors (due to the herbicides themselves or, perhaps more likely, the insecticides that had also been sprayed by this aircraft), so consequently these samples may not be representative of the ORH C-123s in general. The values of samples gathered from the other two C-123s in 2009, however, were quite closely clustered, perhaps an indication of redistribution toward homogeneity on their interior surfaces as they sat sealed on the desert. The only two TCDD air samples collected were collected in 2009 using a screening sampling method (USAF, 2009b), apparently under conditions of artificial mechanical ventilation (Nieman, 2014), and they both were non-detects. It is clear that any estimate of TCDD exposure to C-123 crews based on these meager data will be very uncertain. Nevertheless, the committee worked with these data in an effort to fulfill its charge by gaining at least some perspective on potential exposures.

To assess whether industrial sites require clean-up, it has become common practice to do a "worst-case scenario" evaluation as an initial screening procedure. Assumptions are made in selecting variables for estimation models to be protective of all exposed individuals; that is, they are "conservative." The committee considered this approach as a potential starting point. In light of its charge to provide the VA with a sense of the plausibility of an increase in health problems actually occurring among the AF Reservists who had worked with ORH C-123s, the committee thought it more constructive to limit the inputs used in exploring various exposure models to ranges more likely to reflect the residues and the work experience of the AF Reserve personnel.

Exposure assessors frequently perform computer simulations, or Monte Carlo modeling, in which the exposure model is run repeatedly with values sampled from the theoretical distributions of each input variable. The results of all the iterations produce a distribution of exposure estimates that describes central tendency and variability for the situation in question. Because of the sparse nature of the available sampling results and the committee's instruction to perform a qualitative assessment of exposure, such an intricate approach was not deemed necessary or scientifically credible.

The limitations of the available sampling data (as described previously) make them inadequate for deriving definitive estimates of exposure, but the committee did explore different approaches to quantitative assessment to gain a sense of magnitude and variability for answering its second charge. The committee does not, however, endorse any particular estimates generated in the course of its quantitative explorations, so specific estimation results are not presented in this report.

The committee had defined the sampling results that would be best for any numerical considerations to be interior TCDD wipe samples. Unfortunately, this set of measurements was limited to eight samples from "Patches" (three in 1994 and five in 1995), and seven and nine samples collected in 2009 from two ORH C-123s that had been stored in the desert for many years (see Table 3-3).

The set of guidelines adopted as being most appropriate for comparison with the sampling results were those for surface loadings on indoor surfaces, which ranged from 1 to 25 TEQ ng/m^2 (see Table 2-1). Derived between 1983 and 2009, they seem to have tended toward greater stringency as data and understanding of the toxicity of dioxin-like chemicals increased. They include the 3.5 ng/m^2 screening level derived by CHPPM and the 22 ng/m^2 guideline found in the 2009 AF report (which should have been 1.1 ng/m^2, if dermal exposure had been taken into account as claimed; see Table 4-1). The committee considered this range of surface standards as roughly defining zone in which observation of sampling measurements suggests transition into a level of exposures plausibly associated with consequential increases the risk of health problems.

It was the committee's understanding that the VA's interest is in determining whether the AF Reservists had plausibly been at risk of experiencing exposures hazardous to their heath. With this objective, strict adherence to the public health practice, or "precautionary principle" that adopts very protective assumptions to ensure that no health threat to a population might be overlooked seemed inappropriate to the committee. Therefore, in its efforts to establish the plausible magnitude of the AF Reservists' exposures, the committee considered values reflective of their actual work experience, rather than the extreme or "worst-case" values that are often used in risk assessments. When putting its perceptions of the available data in context, however, the committee accepted international screening guidelines, generally derived in accord with the precautionary principle, as defining a range of values at which taking further action in the interest of health would be merited.

Most of the guidelines that the committee used to put the possible exposures of C-123 personnel in context were developed for hypothetical long-term office workers (an application of the precautionary principle), but information on the work profiles of the AF Reservists was far too unclear to permit adjustment of the guidelines to match their work experience. Although the cumulative time the AF Reservists spent in ORH C-123s was less than 30- to 40-year working lifetimes, the nature of the C-123 personnel's work activities may have increased the exposure experienced per unit of time, thereby reducing the "protectiveness" of the guideline. Also, several of the guidelines expressed in terms of surface TCDD levels do not account for the extent of dermal absorption. While such guidelines are generally derived with the intention of being protective, if the guidelines do not factor in all routes of exposure or activities of the workers, then their tendency toward protectiveness from "worst-case" estimation of risk would be diminished.

The extent to which the levels of TCDD in the aircraft would degrade or be depleted over time was also uncertain. Several committee members thought that the levels of sampled residues would reflect only a small fraction of the concentrations present during the decade of use after the ORH C-123s returned from Vietnam. There was no consensus on the value for the fraction degraded or depleted over time, but all agreed that the contamination at the time of sampling would have been less than it had been at the time of exposure at least 10 years earlier. Therefore, the long delay between the time of exposure and the time of sampling would at worst contribute to underestimation of the AF Reservists' exposure.

In other respects, comparisons of exposure estimates for the AF Reservists to established guidelines are associated with a great deal of uncertainty, but there is no reason to anticipate an overall trend of systematic over- or underestimation of health risks. For example, it was not at all clear that the three sampled planes and the 24 interior samples gathered were representative of the ORH C-123s used by the AF Reservists or the surfaces with which they had contact. Although this is a substantial source of uncertainty, there is no evidence suggesting their selection was biased toward over- or underestimation.

These arguments recognize considerable uncertainty, but they do provide support for concluding that the reported TCDD surface levels are very unlikely to be systematic overestimates in comparison to the existing surface loading guidelines. Table 4-4 is a compilation of sources of uncertainty demonstrating that there are a substantial number that might be expected to tend toward underestimation of the exposures and associated health risks experienced by the AF Reservists, which together may go far toward neutralizing the protective bias normally built into guidelines. Screening guidelines are intended to provide protection for workers with a vast range of far less extreme values than those of the hypothetical office workers used in deriving the guideline.

The committee became convinced that simply comparing the unadjusted surface measurements from the ORH C-123 to the existing guidelines for surface loading provides a valid qualitative means based on international regulatory standards for envisioning the degree of health risk associated with these results (see Figure 4-1).

Given the variety of approaches pursued in its efforts to interpret the available data and the intrinsic weaknesses of those data, the committee was unable to determine which, if any, of the various models and exposure scenarios investigated should be regarded as the most reliable representation of the experiences of the AF Reservists. The committee observed, however, that under at least some reasonable scenario, all the models that were considered generated exposure estimates for the C-123 personnel that were larger than what screening guidelines deemed to be "acceptably" safe. Several factors contributing to uncertainty

TABLE 4-4 Likely Directionality of Various Sources of Uncertainty Involved in Assessing Exposure of AF Reservists Who Used ORH C-123s on the Basis of Available Sampling Results

Source of Uncertainty If Quantitative Exposure Estimates Were Derived from C-123 Surface Sample Data	Direction of Bias in Estimation of Exposure or Risk
Representativeness of sampled aircraft and locations sampled	None perceived
Samples gathered long after the period of potential exposure	Underestimate
Wipe samples may indicate levels that are "substantially below true surface levels" (EPA, 1991)	Underestimate
Air sampling insufficiently sensitive	Underestimate
Degree of uptake from surfaces by the AF Reservists versus assumptions in surface guidelines for office workers	Overall directionality unclear
• Duration in contaminated space—less, but likely also the case for target population of guideline	
• Intensity of physical activity—greater	
• Contact with surfaces—greater	
Exposure estimates in terms of TCDD only versus guidelines in terms of TEQs	Minimal underestimate of total TEQ exposure in case of AO-derived residues
Screening guidelines—"worst-case" approach is designed to be health protective	Generally over estimate risk, but may not be as protective as thought
• Upper limit on potency factor	Protective
• Extreme duration of exposure	Protective
• Failure to incorporate exposure by all routes	Non-protective
• Older guidelines do not include more sensitive TCDD exposure–response information from new research	Non-protective
• Reservists exposed when TEQ burdens were high for general population	Non-protective for threshold effects

NOTES: AF, US Air Force; AO, Agent Orange; ORH, Operation Ranch Hand; TCDD, 2,3,7,8-tetrachlorodibenzo-*p*-dioxin; TEQ, toxicity equivalency quotient.

discussed in this report (such as the long delay between when the activities leading to possible exposure occurred and sampling, the failure to adequately account for the extent of dermal absorption, considering only TCDD measurements in comparison to the screening levels developed in terms of TEQs for all dioxin-like chemicals contributing to exposure overall, etc.) would be expected to bias exposure estimates toward underestimation and hence an understatement of projected risk for the AF Reservists. Such tendencies toward underestimation would countervail to a certain extent against the built-in "worst-case" nature of

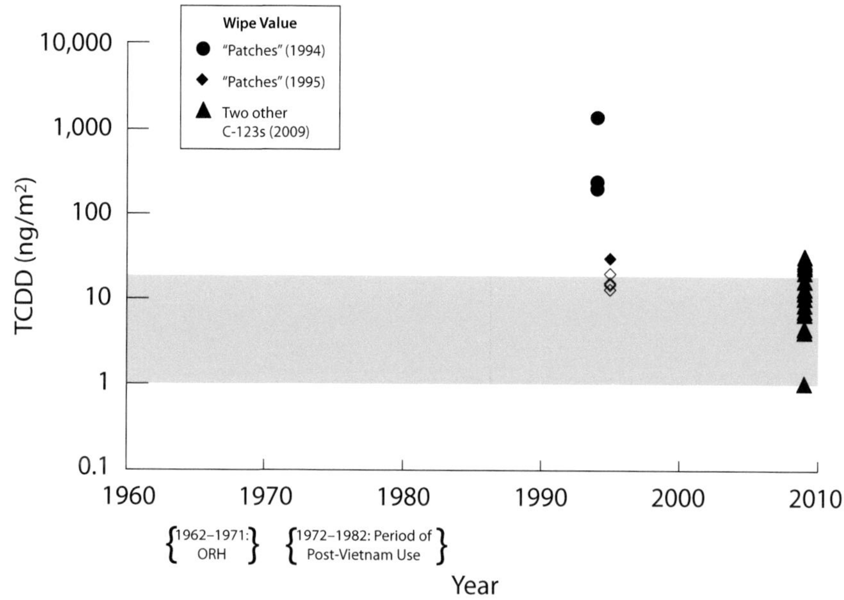

FIGURE 4-1 Existing guidelines for TCDD Surface concentrations in relation to results of interior wipe samples.
NOTE: TCDD surface concentrations obtained from the total of 24 wipe samples from the interiors of post-Vietnam C-123 aircraft by year. The horizontal band represents the 1–25 ng/m^2 range of existing surface guidelines for TCDD. Clear points represent non-detect samples plotted at their detection limit. The concentration of TCDD in four samples gathered from "Patches" in 1994 were below their limits of detection, which in turn were not sensitive enough to evaluate whether or not the samples' concentrations were less than 1 ng/m^2 (below the range of concern).

the available guidelines considered. When even these quite probably understated values fall in the region delineated by the screening levels for interior surfaces derived by several expert regulatory groups, the committee's reasons for attributing plausibility to the occurrence of nontrivial increases in the risk of adverse health outcomes have a firm basis.

5

Summary of Findings

The committee's charge consisted of two tasks:

- Evaluate the reliability (including representativeness, consistency, methods used) of the available information for establishing exposure.
- Address and place in context (qualitatively by comparison to established exposure guidelines) whether any documented residues represent potentially harmful exposure by characterizing the amounts available and the degree to which absorption might be expected.

Some of the desired types of information (particularly ample sampling information from the time of the Reservists' exposure) that any exposure assessor would prefer to have when addressing these tasks simply do not exist. Similarly, much other important information is not available in any definitive form. The committee did its best to integrate the information provided by the military through the US Department of Veterans Affairs (VA), from the retired Air Force (AF) Reservists, and by other interested parties. Relevant publications from the peer-reviewed literature were consulted, but a great many of the critical documents (for example, personal statements, letters, memos, and commissioned reports) fall into the category of documents that have not been peer-reviewed, sometimes referred to as "grey literature," and so must be regarded as being somewhat less than authoritative.

In numerous instances, information and opinions from various sources (documents and people) differed considerably. Controversy about many issues persists with no definitive way to establish what the facts are. The committee is not in a position to make final judgments surrounding discrepancies between the recollections of military personnel and those of the AF Reservists. In some instances, the resolution of these very heated debates would make very little difference in the execution of the committee's task. For instance, this is the case for the dispute about what efforts were made to decontaminate the Operation Ranch Hand (ORH) C-123s before their use by the Reservists or even what decontamination measures were taken by the Reservists themselves. No matter what methods may have been used, TCDD and phenoxy herbicide residues were still detected 30 years later in several of the C-123 aircraft at levels in excess of international guidelines. The committee anchored its deliberations upon the facts available for incorporation in the scientific endeavor of exposure estimation and did not give particular credence to any party's recollection of the events.

The committee notes that the two bulleted tasks in its charge are followed by

> The possible health effects would be assumed to be those characterized in prior Veterans and Agent Orange reports, and would not be re-assessed for this report. VAO activities to date have found the information concerning the exposure of Vietnam Veterans inadequate to establish dose-response relationships for individual health outcomes or to quantify the risk of a particular Veteran experiencing any adverse effect.

This committee does concur with earlier IOM committees responsible for the biennial updates in the Veterans and Agent Orange (VAO) series that there are inadequate data to establish dose–response relationships for particular health outcomes or to quantify the increased risk of any individual veteran to experience any adverse effect. The committee's task has been to assess whether the AF Reservists using the C-123s that had sprayed herbicides in Vietnam had experienced exposures that might increase their risk of ***any*** adverse health outcome. The estimates of toxic potency underlying the guidelines referred to by the committee have been derived from controlled animal studies, rather than the epidemiologic results that underlie conclusions concerning association in the VAO series.

FINDINGS IN RESPONSE TO THE FIRST TASK OF THE COMMITTEE'S CHARGE

Only very limited sampling data were collected from the C-123s, and all but the 1979 herbicide samples from "Patches" were gathered decades after the AF Reservists' exposures on the aircraft had occurred. The data include a series of spot samples in a subset of the planes used by the Reservists with only some of the sampled aircraft having been used in ORH. The limitations of the data available on the levels of TCDD contamination in the interior of the C-123 planes used between 1972 and 1982 by the AF Reservists include the following:

- The sampling efforts were not designed to quantitatively assess the potential exposure to the AF Reservists.

- TCDD sampling was not contemporaneous with the exposure period of concern, and there is great uncertainty about what changes in TCDD levels had occurred inside the planes, during active use prior to 1982 when depletion due to high air turnover would have been maximal and then during their long storage in the desert.
- Sampling and analysis methods used over the various sampling periods apparently were not uniform, but the methodologies were not fully described. Aside from the air samples which were collected using inappropriate methods, however, the committee did not find information to invalidate any of the reported measurement data.
- Considerable nonuniformity in the distribution of contamination throughout the interior of "Patches" and differences in sampling procedures may have contributed to the inconsistencies noted between the sampling results in 1994 and 1995.
- Detailed, reliable information is not available on the activities of aircrews and maintenance personnel inside these airplanes (e.g., time spent in planes, contacts with surfaces, use of protective equipment, etc.) and very little information is available on the use of specific aircraft.
- The limitations of the available information make them inadequate for deriving definitive quantitative estimates of exposure, but they are sufficient for a screening level of analysis. Despite these limitations, it is significant that the interiors of the C-123s that had sprayed herbicides in Vietnam and were later used by the AF Reservists had Agent Orange (AO) and TCDD contamination at levels in excess of international guidelines long after their use by the AF Reserve personnel.

Understanding of the physical and chemical characteristics of semi-volatile organic compounds (SVOCs) like TCDD establishes that they would not be immobilized on surfaces, so residues were available for transfer by dermal contact, inhalation, and ingestion. AF Reservists serving in the contaminated C-123s, therefore, experienced some degree of exposure to TCDD and herbicides through multiple routes when working in ORH C-123s. The committee notes that the sampling results appear to be consistent with redistribution of dioxin in accordance with established thermodynamic principles which predict more uniform readings as contamination in hot spots vaporize and resettle averaging out the concentration over the entire interior surface with the passage of time. The exposure potential of individuals working in that environment was likely highly variable. Even if the sampling results were considered an adequate basis for estimating exposure, the information necessary for derivation of estimates on an individual basis is not available.

Air TCDD levels would be expected to be higher on the ground than while flying, due to lower air circulation. Maintenance workers would, therefore, be expected to have higher inhalation exposures per time spent in the planes than crew members. Work practices of maintenance workers may also have involved more contact with contaminated surfaces than those of crew members. Consequently, depending on the amount of time maintenance workers spent in planes, their TCDD exposures could have been higher than those of C-123 crew members.

FINDINGS IN RESPONSE TO THE SECOND TASK OF THE COMMITTEE'S CHARGE

- Of the various interpretations of the available data available for review, the committee finds the Agency for Toxic Substances and Disease Registry's (ATSDR's) qualitative assessment (2012, 2013a,b, 2014) to be the most reasonable and well-supported.
- How representative the very limited number of TCDD samples gathered from the ORH C-123s are of the TCDD distribution throughout their interior is uncertain, but, in the absence of definitive information to the contrary, the committee assumed that the three ORH C-123s sampled were representative of the entire fleet.
- There is no definitive information on the rate of degradation or depletion of TCDD on interior surfaces of the aircraft in the decades after their use in ORH. Without adjustment for reductions in the contamination over time, estimates of TCDD exposures to the AF Reservists based on samples taking from the C-123s in the mid-1990s and in 2009 could, therefore, underestimate their actual exposures, quite possibly markedly. Therefore, the measurements resulting from interior surface sampling in 1994, 1995, and 2009 probably represent a lower bound on what average surface TCDD contamination might have been when the AF Reservists worked in the planes.
- Because of problems related to factoring dermal absorption into the some guidelines, the committee recognized that several of those referred to during its evaluation might not be as protective as supposed. Several guidelines underestimated the extent to which dermal absorption contributes to total exposure in the workplace. In another instance, a guideline for surface loading purported to be protective for the combination of dermal and oral exposure was calculated erroneously so that the more sensitive dermal pathway effectively had not been factored in.
- The committee did not find any of the existing contamination guidelines for TCDD it reviewed or the three models as presented and parameterized in Lurker et al. (2014) a perfect match for the circumstances being evaluated, but it did decide that the surface Toxicity Equivalency Quotient (TEQ) loading guidelines were most applicable to the AF Reservist's occupational situation.
- The committee switched its attentions to the guidelines themselves after determining that efforts to adjust the poorly documented work profiles of

the Reservists to correspond with those hypothesized for office workers in deriving the guideline had an indeterminate effect. It is the committee's judgment that comparing the unadjusted surface measurements from the ORH C-123s to the existing guidelines for surface loading provides the most valid qualitative means of evaluating the degree to which these results accord with international guidelines.

- The existing guidelines for TEQs on interior surfaces ranged from 1 to 25 ng/m^2, demarcating a zone in which sampling measurements reach a level where action should be taken.

Although the existing information is inadequate for estimating exposure with any degree of certainty, the committee was able to answer its charge to evaluate the reliability of the data and to qualitatively establish whether the documented residues represent potentially harmful exposures.

The available sampling data are sufficient to demonstrate long-term Agent Orange and TCDD contamination of the C-123s. Understanding of the physical and chemical properties of TCDD establishes that residues measured on the inorganic surfaces within the C-123s would not have been immobile and that contact with the exterior of the AF Reservists' bodies would have occurred to some extent. Retrospective estimation of concentrations present at the time of the AF Reservists' service based on these limited measurements would inevitably be subject to substantial uncertainty. At the time when the AF Reservists were working on these C-123s, the levels of TCDD would have been at least as high as those measured at later times. Hence, exposure estimates based on the collected samples without adjustment for any depletion of the TCDD loading on interior surfaces would likely underestimate the actual exposure experienced many years earlier. Direct comparison of those surface loading measurements with existing TCDD guidelines without additional adjustments to incorporate assumptions about work practices during stateside use of the ORH C-123s would not be expected to systematically overestimate their exposures and associated risks.

Bearing in mind all of the factors discussed above, the committee reached consensus that it is probable that the TCDD exposures of at least some AF Reservists exceeded levels equivalent to some guidelines established for office workers in enclosed settings. The committee's interpretation of the available data is that, although they do not permit definitive quantitative estimation of exposure due to a multitude of uncertainties, they do indicate that it is plausible that the C-123s did contribute to some adverse health consequences among the AF Reservists who worked in ORH C-123s after the planes returned from Vietnam. The committee is firm in its conviction that the AF Reservists working in ORH C-123s were exposed (in the technical sense of the word of having bodily contact with the chemicals) to the components of AO to some extent. The committee members could not stand behind any particular exposure estimates produced by manipulating the existing data, but they are clear in their finding that the surface-wipe sampling measurements of dioxin gathered in 1994, 1995, and 2009 are fully consistent with exposures to the AF Reservists while working in ORH C-123 planes that exceeded international exposure guidelines.

Of the ORH C-123s returned to the United States from Vietnam, most have been destroyed. The exceptions are the now decontaminated C-123 at Wright-Patterson Air Force Base and two other C-123s that did go to Vietnam and most probably sprayed herbicides (although documentation remains lacking) are on display at military aviation museums in Delaware and Georgia (the public is not permitted access to their interiors). Efforts to recover the work records of the AF Reservists have been unsuccessful, so it is highly unlikely that any additional information will become available to establish more definitively the magnitude of exposures experienced by the AF Reservists.

References

AF Working Paper (Air Force Working Paper). 1979. Protocol, Project Ranch Hand II–Epidemiologic Investigation of Health Effects in Air Force Personnel Following Exposure to "Herbicide Orange." USAF School of Aerospace Medicine, Brooks Air Force Base, Texas (December 12).

AFHS (Air Force Health Study). 1982. *An epidemiologic investigation of health effects in Air Force personnel following exposure to herbicides: Study protocol, initial report*. Brooks AFB, TX: USAF School of Aerospace Medicine. SAM-TR-82-44.

AFHS. 1983. *An epidemiologic investigation of health effects in Air Force personnel following exposure to herbicides*. Baseline Mortality Study Results. Brooks AFB, TX: USAF School of Aerospace Medicine. NTIS AD-A130 793.

AFHS. 1991. *An epidemiologic investigation of health effects in Air Force personnel following exposure to herbicides*. Serum Dioxin Analysis of 1987 Examination Results. Brooks AFB, TX: USAF School of Aerospace Medicine. AL-TR-91-0009.

AFHS. 1995. *An epidemiologic investigation of health effects in Air Force personnel following exposure to herbicides*. 1992 Follow-up Examination Results. Brooks AFB, TX: Epidemiologic Research Division. Armstrong Laboratory. AL-TR-920107.

AFHS. 2000. *An epidemiologic investigation of health effects in Air force personnel following exposure to herbicides*. 1997 Follow-up Examination Results. Brooks AFB, TX: Human Systems Program Office. Armstrong Laboratory. AFRL-HE-BR-TR-2000-02.

AFHS. 2005. *An epidemiologic investigation of health effects in Air Force personnel following exposure to herbicides*. 2002 Follow-up Examination Results. Brooks AFB, TX: Epidemiologic Research Division. Armstrong Laboratory. AFRL-HE-BR-SR-2005-0003.

AMARG (309th Aerospace Maintenance and Regeneration Group). 2014. *What is AMARG?* http://www.amarcexperience.com/ui/index.php?option=com_content&view=article&id=2&Itemid=213 (accessed July 31, 2014).

ATSDR (Agency for Toxic Substances and Disease Registry). 1998. *Toxicological profile for chlorinated dibenzo*-p-*dioxins*. http://www.atsdr.cdc.gov/toxprofiles/tp104.pdf (accessed July 20, 2014).

ATSDR. 2012. Letter from Thomas Sinks, Deputy Director, National Center for Environmental Health and ATSDR to Major Wesley Carter. January 25, 2012.

ATSDR. 2013a. Letter from Christopher J. Portier, Director, National Center, and Environmental Health, ATSDR to Domenic A. Baldini Chief, Joint Services Records Research Center US Army Records Management and Declassification Agency. March 6, 2013.

ATSDR. 2013b. Letter from Robin M. Ikeda, Deputy Director, Noncommunicable Disease, Injury, and Environmental Health Acting Director, National Center for Environmental Health/ATSDR to Major Wesley Carter. March 6, 2013.

ATSDR. 2014. Exposure Modeling with Existing Data. Slide presentation from Thomas Sinks to the Committee to Evaluate the Potential Exposure to Agent Orange/TCDD Residue and Level of Risk of Adverse Health Effects for Aircrew of Post-Vietnam C-123 Aircraft. June 16, 2014.

Battista, A. B. 2014. Letter to the Committee to Evaluate the Potential Exposure to Agent Orange/ TCDD Residue and Level of Risk of Adverse Health Effects for Aircrew of Post-Vietnam C-123 Aircraft: A C-123K Pilot's Perspective. June 12, 2014.

Bennett, D. H., and E. J. Furtaw Jr. 2004. Fugacity-based indoor residential pesticide fate model. *Environmental Science and Technology* 38(7):2142–2152.

Berman, F. 2011. Letter from Fred Berman, Director, CROET Toxicology Information Center, Center for Research on Occupational and Environmental Toxicology, Oregon Health and Science University to the Secretary of the Air Force and Veterans of the C-123K Provider Who Served Between 1972–1982. May 25, 2011.

California EPA (Environmental Protection Agency). 1999. *Chronic toxicity summary: Chlorinated dibenzo-*p*-dioxins and chlorinated dibenzofurans (including 2,3,7,8-tetrachlorodibenzo-*p*-dioxin).* Office of Environmental Health Hazard Assessment. http://oehha.ca.gov/air/chronic_rels/pdf/chlordibenz.pdf (accessed July 20, 2014).

Carter, W. 2013. *Decades of deception, 1971–2013—C-123 veterans: VA illegally denies Agent Orange claims.* C-123 Veterans Administration. McMinnville, OR.

Carter, W. 2014a. C-123 Veteran statement regarding questions raised, and answers #102. Department of Veterans Affairs, Statement in Support of Claim, June 29.

Carter, W. 2014b. Responses to IOM questions. Workshop submission on behalf of the C-123 Veterans Association (Personal correspondence, June 16).

CDC (Centers for Disease Control). 1988. Serum 2,3,7,8-tetrachlorodibenzo-*p*-dioxin levels in US Army Vietnam era veterans. *Journal of the American Medical Association* 260:1249–1254.

Cecil, P. F. 1986. *Herbicidal warfare: The Ranch Hand Project.* New York: Praeger Special Studies, Praeger Scientific.

Cecil, P. F., and A. L. Young. 2008. Operation FLYSWATTER: A war within a war. *Environmental Science and Pollution Research* 15(1):3–7.

CHPPM (US Army Center for Health Promotion and Preventive Medicine). 2009. *Technical guide 312: Health risk assessment methods and screening levels for evaluating office worker exposures to contaminants on indoor surfaces using surface wipe data.* USACHPPM TG-312. Aberdeen Proving Ground, MD.

Courtney, K. D., D. W. Gaylor, M. D. Hogan, H. L. Falk, R. R. Bates, and I. Mitchel. 1970. Teratogenic evaluation of 2,4,5-T. *Science* 168(3933):864–866.

Deziel, N. C., S. M. Viet, J. W. Rogers, D. E. Camann, D. A. Marker, M. S. A. Heikkinen, A. Y. Yau, D. M. Stout, and M. Dellarco. 2011. Comparison of wipe materials and wetting agents for pesticide residue collection from hard surfaces. *Science for the Total Environment* 409:4442–4448.

Driver, J. H., and K. Solomon. 2014. Comments to the IOM Committee Regarding Exposure Modelling in the Paper "Lurker PA, Berman F, Clapp RW, Stellman JM. 2014. Post-Vietnam military herbicide exposures in UC-123 Agent Orange spray aircraft. *Environmental Research* 130:34–42."

EC (European Commission, Scientific Committee on Food). 2001. *Opinion of the Scientific Committee on Food on the risk assessment of dioxins and dioxin-like PCBs in food. Updated opinion based on new scientific information available since the adoption of the SCF opinion of 22 November 2000. Adopted on 30 May 2001*, CS/CNTM/DIOXIN/20 Final. Brussels: European Commission, Scientific Committee on Food. http://ec.europa.eu/food/fs/sc/scf/out90_en.pdf (accessed July 20, 2014).

EPA (US Environmental Protection Agency). 1989. *Risk assessment guidance for Superfund Volume I: Human health evaluation manual (Part A): Interim final*. Office of Emergency and Remedial Response. EPA/540/1-89/002. December 1989. http://www.epa.gov/oswer/riskassessment/ragsa (accessed May 22, 2014).

EPA. 1991. *Wipe sampling and double wash/rinse cleanup as recommended by Environmental Protection Agency PCB Spill Cleanup Policy.* June 23, 1987—Revised and Clarified on April 18, 1991. US Environmental Protection Agency, Washington, DC.

EPA. 1992. *National primary drinking water regulations, technical factsheet on: Dioxin (2,3,7,8-TCDD)*. Finalized July 1992. http://www.epa.gov/ogwdw/pdfs/factsheets/soc/tech/dioxin.pdf (accessed May 22, 2014).

EPA. 2000. *Benchmark dose technical guidance document* (External Review Draft). EPA/630/R-00/001.

EPA. 2001. *General principles for performing aggregate exposure and risk assessments.* Office of Pesticide Programs, US Environmental Protection Agency, Washington, DC, Item 6043.

EPA. 2012. *EPA's reanalysis of key issues related to dioxin toxicity and response to NAS Comments, Volume 1: In support of summary information on the Integrated Risk Information System (IRIS)* EPA/600/R-10/038F. US Environmental Protection Agency, Washington, DC.

Ertl, H., and W. Butte. 2012. Bioaccessibility of pesticides and polychlorinated biphenyls from house dust: *In-vitro* methods and human exposure. *Journal of Exposure Science and Environmental Epidemiology* 22:574–583.

German MAK-Wert (guideline set in 1999 with documentation in German); published online (January 31, 2012) by The Wiley Online Library as part of The MAK Collection for Occupational Health and Safety. http://onlinelibrary.wiley.com/doi/10.1002/3527600418.mb174601d0028/pdf (accessed July 20, 2014).

Gravitz, N., A. Fan, and R. R. Neutra. 1983. *Interim guidelines for acceptable exposure levels in office settings contaminated with PCB and PCB combustion products*. Epidemiological Studies Section, California Department of Health Services.

Harris, S. A., and K. R. Solomon. 1992. Percutaneous penetration of 2,4-dichlorophenoxyacetic acid and 2,4-D dimethylamine salt in human volunteers. *Journal of Toxicology and Environmental Health* 36(3):233–220.

IOM (Institute of Medicine). 1994. *Veterans and Agent Orange: Health effects of herbicides used in Vietnam*. Washington, DC: National Academy Press.

IOM. 2009. *Veterans and Agent Orange: Update 2008*. Washington, DC: The National Academies Press.

IOM. 2011. *Blue Water Navy Vietnam Veterans and Agent Orange Exposure*. Washington, DC: The National Academies Press.

IOM. 2012. *Veterans and Agent Orange: Update 2010*. Washington, DC: The National Academies Press.

IOM. 2014. *Veterans and Agent Orange: Update 2012*. Washington, DC: The National Academies Press.

Japanese EA (Japanese Environmental Agency). 1999. *Report on tolerable daily intake (TDI) of dioxins and related compounds (Japan)*. Environmental Health Committee of the Central Environment Council Environment Agency, Living Environment Council and Food Sanitation Investigation Council Ministry of Health and Welfare. 53 pp.

Johansson, N., and A. Hanberg. 2000. Report from a Nordic meeting on the 1998 WHO consultation on assessment of the health risks of dioxins; Re-evaluation of the tolerable daily intake (TDI). *Organohalogen Compounds* 48:252–255.

Karch, N. J., D. K. Watkins, A. L. Young, and M. E. Ginevan. 2004. Environmental fate of TCDD and Agent Orange and bioavailability to troops in Vietnam. *Organohalogen Compounds* 66:3689–3694.

Kerger, B., G. Corbett, S. El-Sururi, R. Reitz, and D. Paustenbach. 1995. Validating Dermal Exposure Assessment Techniques for Dioxin Using Body Burden Data and Pharmacokinetic Modeling. *Organohalogen Compounds* 25:137–142.

Kim, N. K., and J. Hawley. 1985. *Re-entry Guidelines: Binghamton State Office Building*. Bureau of Toxic Substance Assessment, Division of Environmental Health Assessment, New York State Department of Health: Albany, NY.

Kimbrough, R. D., C. A. Krouskas, M. L. Carson, T. F. Long, C. Bevan, and R. G. Tardiff. 2010. Human uptake of persistent chemicals from contaminated soil: PCDD/Fs and PCBs. *Regulatory Toxicology and Pharmacology* 57(1):43–54.

Kissel, J. C. 2011. The mismeasure of dermal absorption. *Journal of Exposure Science and Environmental Epidemiology* 21(3):302–309.

Lees, P. S. J., M. Corn, and P. N. Breysse. 1987. Evidence for dermal absorption as the major route of body entry during exposure of transformer maintenance and repairmen to PCBs. *American Industrial Hygiene Association Journal* 48(3):257–264.

Liang, Y., and Y. Xu. 2014. Improved method for measuring and characterizing phthalate emissions from building materials and its application to exposure assessment. *Environmental Science and Technology* 48:4475–4484.

Lindquist, N. G., and S. Ullberg. 1971. Distribution of the herbicides 2,4,5-T and 2,4-D in pregnant mice: Accumulation in the yolk sac epithelium. *Experientia* 27(12):1439–1441.

Little, J. C., C. J. Weschler, W. W. Nazaroff, Z. Liu, and E. A. Cohen Hubal. 2012. Rapid methods to estimate potential exposure to semivolatile organic compounds in the indoor environment. *Environmental Science and Technology* 46(20):11171–11178.

Liu, Q. T., R. Chen, B. E. McCarry, M. L. Diamond, and B. Bahavar. 2003. Characterizaion of polar organic compounds in the organic film on indoor and outdoor glass windows. *Environmental Science and Technology* 37(11):2340–2349.

Lurker, P. A., F. Berman, R. W. Clapp, J. M. Stellman. 2014. Post-Vietnam military herbicide exposures in UC-123 Agent Orange spray aircraft. *Environmental Research* 130:34–42.

Mackay, D. 2001. *Multimedia environmental models: The fugacity approach*, 2nd ed. Boca Raton, FL: Lewis Publishers.

May, L. M., B. Gaborek, T. Pitrat, and L. Peters. 2002. Derivation of risk based wipe surface screening levels for industrial scenarios. *Science of the Total Environment* 288(1–2):65–80.

McGregor, D. B., C. Partenski, J. Wilbourn, and J. M. Rice. 1998. An IARC evaluation of polychlorinated dibenzo-*p*-dioxins and polychlorinated dibenzofurans as risk factors in human carcinogenesis. *Environmental Health Perspectives* 106(S2):775–760.

Meek, S. L. 1981. *An estimate of the relative exposure of U.S. Air Force crewmembers to Agent Orange*. Master thesis, University of Washington.

Melius, J. 1985. Letter from PCB Expert Advisory Panel to the Honorable Tony Anaya, Governor of the State of New Mexico. (As cited in NRC, 1988.)

Michalek, J. E., and M. Pavuk. 2008. Diabetes and cancer in veterans of Operation Ranch Hand after adjustment for calendar period, days of spraying, and time spent in Southeast Asia. *Journal of Occupational and Environmental Medicine* 50(3):330–340.

Michalek, J. E., W. H. Wolfe, J. C. Miner, T. M. Papa, and J. L. Pirkle. 1995. Indices of TCDD exposure and TCDD body burden in veterans of Operation Ranch Hand. *Journal of Exposure Analysis and Environmental Epidemiology* 5(2):209–223.

Mocarelli, P., P. M. Gerthoux, D. G. Patterson Jr., S. Milani, G. Limonta, M. Bertona, S. Signorini, P. Tramacere, L. Colombo, C. Crespi, P. Brambilla, C. Sarto, V. Carreri, E. J. Sampson, W. E. Turner, and L .L Needham. 2008. Dioxin exposure, from infancy through puberty, produces endocrine disruption and affects human semen quality. *Environmental Health Perspectives* 116(1):70–77.

Moody, R. P., C. A. Franklin, L. Ritter, and H. I. Maibach. 1990. Dermal absorption of the phenoxy herbicides 2,4-D, 2,4-D amine, 2,4-D isooctyl, and 2,4,5-T in rabbits, rats, rhesus monkeys, and humans: A cross-species comparison. *Journal of Toxicology and Environmental Health* 29(3):237–245. Erratum in *Journal of Toxicology and Environmental Health* 32(1):107–108, 1991.

MRI (Midwest Research Institute). 1967. *Assessment of Ecological Effects of Extensive or Repeated Use of Herbicides*. MRI Project No. 3103-B. Kansas City, MO: MRI. NTIS AD-824-314.

NIEHS (National Institute of Environmental Health Sciences). 2011. Letter from Linda S. Birnbaum, Director, NIEHS and National Toxicology Program to Major Wesley Carter. June 9, 2011.

NIEHS. 2013. Letter from Aubrey K. Miller, Senior Medical Officer, NIEHS to Major Wesley Carter. March 1, 2013.

Nieman, J. K. C. 2014. Commentary on "Post-Vietnam military herbicide exposures in UC-123 Agent Orange spray aircraft." *Environmental Research* 131:217–218.

NIOSH (National Institute for Occupational Safety and Health). 1991. Dioxin Registry Report of the Dow Chemical Company, Midland, Michigan, Report No. IWS 117.15. Cincinnati, OH. Pp. 43–45.

NRC (National Research Council). 1974. *The effects of herbicides in South Vietnam*. Washington, DC: National Academy Press.

NRC. 1988. *Acceptable levels of dioxin contamination in an office building following a transformer fire*. Washington, DC: National Academy Press.

Poiger, H., and C. Schlatter. 1980. Influence of solvents and adsorbents on dermal and intestinal absorption of TCDD. *Food and Cosmetics Toxicology* 18(5):477–481.

RIVM (Rijksinstituut voor Volksgezondheid en Milieu). 2001. *Re-evaluation of human-toxicological maximum permissible risk levels.* Chapter 5.12 Dioxins, furans and dioxin-like PCBs (evaluated in 1999), RIVM Report 711701 025. Bilthoven: Dutch National Institute of Public Health and the Environment. http://www.rivm.nl/bibliotheek/rapporten/711701025.html (accessed June 19, 2014). (As cited in UKEA, 2009.)

Robinson, J. N., K. A. Fox, W. G. Jackson, N. S. Ketchum, M. Pavuk, and W. Grubbs. 2006. Air Force Health Study: An Overview. *Organohalogen Compounds* 68:752–755.

Schecter, A. 2013. Letter from Arnold Schecter, Professor, Environmental and Occupational Health Program, University of Texas School of Public Health to Major Wesley Carter. January 2, 2013.

Slayton, T. M., P. A. Valberg, and A. D. Wait. 1998. Estimating dermal transfer from PCB-contaminated porous surfaces. *Chemosphere* 36(14):3003–3014.

Stellman, J. M. 2012. Letter from Jeanne M. Stellman, Professor Emerita and Special Lecturer, Columbia University to Major Wesley Carter. February 7, 2012.

Stellman, J. M. 2013. Letter from Jeanne M. Stellman, Professor Emerita and Special Lecturer, Columbia University to Brigadier General Allison Hickey, Undersecretary for Benefits, Department of Veterans Affairs. November 29, 2013.

Stellman, J. M., S. D. Stellman, R. Christian, T. Weber, and C. Tomasallo. 2003. The extent and patterns of usage of Agent Orange and other herbicides in Vietnam. *Nature* 422(6933):681–687.

UKEA (Environment Agency of the United Kingdom). 2009. *Contaminants in soil: Updated collation of toxicological data and intake values for humans; dioxins, furans, and dioxin-like PCBs.* Science Report: SC050021/TOX 12, Better Regulation Sciences Programme.

USAF (US Department of the Air Force). 1979. *Aircraft Sampling, Westover AFB*. Technical Report No. 79-59, USAF Occupational and Environmental Health Laboratory, Brooks AFB, TX (September 1979).

USAF. 1994. Memo to 645 MedGrp/SGB; Consultative Letter, AL/OE-CL-1994-0203, *Review of dioxin sampling results from C-123 Aircraft, Wright Patterson AFB, OH and recommendations for protection of aircraft restoration personnel.* U.S. Department of the Air Force, Brooks AFB, TX.

USAF. 1995a. *Wipe samples from C123 cargo plane Wright Patterson Air Force Base, Aviation Museum Annex, WPAFB, Ohio.* Analytical Report, Task Order 95-15, Contract F33601-93-DW017. OHM Remediation Services Corporation.

USAF. 1995b. *Appendix A: Wipe samples from C123 cargo plane Wright Patterson Air Force Base, Aviation Museum Annex, WPAFB, Ohio.* Analytical Report, Task Order 95-15, Contract F33601-93-DW017. OHM Remediation Services Corporation.

USAF. 1995c. *Appendix B: Wipe samples from C123 cargo plane Wright Patterson Air Force Base, Aviation Museum Annex, WPAFB, Ohio.* Analytical Report, Task Order 95-15, Contract F33601-93-DW017. OHM Remediation Services Corporation.

USAF. 1996. Cover letter and sample results from Alta Analytical Laboratory. Alta Batch I.D. 2795. (September 6).

USAF. 1997a. Memorandum for ASAFM/MUC. Employee and Public Access to the C-123 "Patches." (February 26).

USAF. 1997b. Consultative Letter, AL/OE-CL-1997-0053, Cleanup of contaminated aircraft, Aerospace Regeneration Center (Department of Defense, Armstrong Laboratory—Memorandum for HQ AFMC/SGC, Logistics Avenue, Suite 23, Wright Patterson AFB, OH); Attention: Maj Gemperle (March 18).

USAF. 2009a. *Final: US-123K sampling and analysis plan.* Hill AFB, UT.

USAF. 2009b. *Final-dioxin and herbicide characterization of UC-123K Aircraft—Phase 1.* Select Engineering Services, Hill AFB, UT.

USAF. 2009c. Response to comments from Jim Malmgren's presentation on UC-123 disposal given at the Air Force Strike Board meeting at AMARG on 18 June 2009 (Memo for the record).

USAF. 2009d. Spreadsheet leading to Table 1 in Appendix F of USAF (2009b)—Surface Contam Levels rev 1.

USAF. 2012a. *Consultative letter, AFRL-SA-WP-CL-2012-0052, UC-123 Agent Orange exposure assessment, post-Vietnam (1972–1982).* USAF School of Aerospace Medicine, Wright-Patterson AFB, OH.

USAF. 2012b. Memorandum: *Post Vietnam C-123 aircraft Agent Orange exposure.* (Department of Defense, Memorandum from HQ USAF/SG, Washington, DC.

VA (US Department of Veterans Affairs). 2014. *Scientific review of Agent Orange in C-123 aircraft.* http://www.publichealth.va.gov/exposures/agentorange/locations/residue-c123-aircraft/scientific-review.asp (accessed March 11, 2014).

Wallace, L. A., W. R. Ott, and C. J. Weschler. 2014. Ultrafine particles from electric appliances and cooking pans: Experiments suggesting desorption/nucleation of sorbed organics as the primary source. *Indoor Air* 1–11.

Weschler, C. J., and W. W. Nazaroff. 2008. Semivolatile organic compounds in indoor environments. *Atmospheric Environment* 42(40):9018–9040.

Weschler, C. J., and W. W. Nazaroff. 2012. SVOC exposure indoors: Fresh look at dermal pathways. *Indoor Air* 22(5):356–377.

WHO (World Health Organization). 2002a. *Evaluation of certain food additives and contaminants.* Fifty-seventh report of the Joint FAO/WHO Expert Committee on Food Additives. WHO Technical Report Series 909. Geneva: World Health Organization. http://whqlibdoc.who.int/trs/WHO_TRS_909.pdf (accessed April 22, 2014).

WHO. 2002b. *Safety evaluation of certain food additives and contaminants. Polychlorinated dibenzodioxins, polychlorinated dibenzofurans and coplanar polychlorinated biphenyls.* WHO Food Additive Series 48. Geneva: World Health Organization. http://www.inchem.org/documents/jecfa/jecmono/v48je20.htm. (As cited in UKEA, 2009.)

WTC (World Trade Center Indoor Air Task Force Working Group, Contaminants of Potential Concern Committee, and US Environmental Protection Agency, Region II). 2003. *World Trade Center indoor environment assessment: Selecting contaminants of potential concern and setting health-based benchmarks*. New York: US Environmental Protection Agency, Risk Ranking Work Group, Region 2.

Young, A. L. 2009. *The history, use, disposition and environmental fate of Agent Orange*. New York: Springer Science and Business Media, LLC.

Young, A. L. 2014. *A presentation to the Institute of Medicine.* Slide presentation to the Committee to Evaluate the Potential Exposure to Agent Orange/TCDD Residue and Level of Risk of Adverse Health Effects for Aircrew of Post-Vietnam C-123 Aircraft. June 16, 2014.

Young, A. L., and M. Newton. 2004. Long overlooked historical information on Agent Orange and TCDD following massive applications of 2,4,5-T-containing herbicides, Eglin AFB, FL. *Environmental Science and Pollution Research* 11(4):209–221.

Young, A. L., and G. M. Reggiani (Eds.). 1988. *Agent Orange and its Associated Dioxin: Assessment of a Controversy*. Amsterdam: Elsevier.

Young, A. L., and K. L. Young. 2012. *Investigations into the allegations of Agent Orange/dioxin exposure from former Ranch Hand aircraft.* Agent Orange Investigative Report Series, No. 2, November. Department of Veterans Affairs contract #VA-101-12-C-0006.

Young, A. L., and K. L. Young. 2013a. *Discussion points supporting compensation service's position on the UC-123-K claims.* Agent Orange Briefs: Special Topics, Brief No. 1, August 21. Department of Veterans Affairs contract #VA-101-12-C-0006.

Young, A. L., and K. L. Young. 2013b. *Investigations into the allegations concerning 2,4,5-T herbicide.* Agent Orange Investigative Report Series, No. 6, March. Department of Veterans Affairs contract #VA-101-12-C-0006.

Young, A. L., and K. L. Young. 2014a. *Supplement to investigative report: New information on former UC-123K Post-Vietnam issue*. Agent Orange Investigative Report Series, No. 17. May/June. Department of Veterans Affairs contract #VA-101-12-C-0006.

Young, A. L., and K. L. Young. 2014b. *Discussion of the presentation to the Institute of Medicine on C-123K exposure issues*. Agent Orange Briefs: Special Topics, Brief No. 6, June 30. Department of Veterans Affairs contract #VA-101-12-C-0006.

Young A. L., J. A. Calcagni, C. E. Thalken, and J. W. Tremblay. 1978. *The toxicology, environmental fate, and human risk of Herbicide Orange and its associated dioxin*. Technical Report USAF OEHL TR-78-92, USAF Occupational and Environmental Health Laboratory, Aerospace Medical Division, Brooks AFB, TX.

Appendix A

Public Agendas from Committee Meetings

FIRST PUBLIC MEETING
May 15, 2014
Keck Building, Room 106
500 Fifth Street, NW
Washington, DC 20001

1:00 p.m.	Welcome; Goals and Conduct of the Public Meeting; Introduction of Committee Members Robert Herrick, Committee Chair
1:05 p.m.	Charge to the Committee Loren Erickson, US Department of Veterans Affairs (VA)
1:25 p.m.	Major Wesley T. Carter (retired), Chair, C-123 Veterans Association
1:45 p.m.	Other Comments, as Requested by Attendees, and Discussion
2:00 p.m.	Close Public Session

SECOND PUBLIC MEETING/WORKSHOP*
June 16, 2014
Keck Building, Room 100
500 Fifth Street, NW
Washington, DC 20001

Welcome, Goals, Conduct of Meeting, Introduction of Committee Members

8:30 a.m. Robert Herrick, Committee Chair

Panel 1: Post-Vietnam Handling and Use of the C-123s

8:45 a.m. Wesley Carter, C-123 Veterans Association
8:50 a.m. Alvin L. Young, A.L. Young Consulting, Inc.
8:55 a.m. Comments and Questions from Committee Members

Panel 2: Collection and Analysis of Samples

9:45 a.m. Peter Lurker, Germantown Consultants, LLC
9:50 a.m. Peter C. Kahn, AESOP, Rutgers University
9:55 a.m. Thomas E. McKone, University of California, Berkeley
10:00 a.m. Comments and Questions from Committee Members

10:45 a.m. BREAK

Panel 3: Exposure Modeling with Existing Data

11:00 a.m. Thomas H. Sinks, Deputy Director of NCEH, ATSDR
11:05 a.m. Jeanne M. Stellman, Columbia University
11:10 a.m. Patrick Finley, Sandia National Laboratories
11:15 a.m. Jeffrey H. Driver, RiskScience.net
11:20 a.m. Comments and Questions from Committee Members

12:15 p.m. LUNCH

Interpretations of Resulting Exposure Estimates and General Discussion

1:00 p.m. Comments and Questions from Attendees
(Make request to staff for a 5-minute slot before lunch)
1:15 p.m. Additional Comments and Questions from Committee Members
1:30 p.m. General Discussion
2:30 p.m. Adjourn Open Session

---

*Invited meeting participants were asked to make presentations to the committee in response to the following questions:

Post-Vietnam Handling and Use of the C-123s

- What were the methods of cleaning, painting, etc., performed on the C-123s that had sprayed herbicides before they were provided to the Air Force Reserve? How and with what?

- While they were being used by the Air Force (AF) Reservists? Particularly for "Patches"? How frequently were the aircraft cleaned? How and with what?
- What was the usual duration of crew members being inside the C-123s (both in flight and on the ground such as training exercises)? Please include preparation time for a flight, flight time and unloading time. And, what would be a plausible range of time (in hours or parts of an hour) spent in/on the planes? On a single weekend? Over the summer weeks?
- Was any food consumed during a flight, and if so what type and how often?
- What type of activities (on the ground and in the air) were crew members involved in while using the C-123s? (e.g., activities that might result in contact with surfaces, generate dust, exposure to new areas, clean surfaces)—Please estimate the duration of each activity.
- How were the reservists assigned to the airplanes? (e.g., always flying the same planes? Or different assignments made each time? etc.)
- What protective clothing (e.g., gloves, shirts, pants) were worn by pilots, other flight crew, and maintenance personnel when in an aircraft? Did this change seasonally? What facilities were available for cleaning hands within the aircraft?

Collection and Analysis of Samples

- What would be the effect of environmental factors (e.g., sunlight, heat, etc.) on 2,3,7,8-tetrachlorodibenzo-*p*-dioxin (TCDD) degradation? Are there other factors that might affect degradation? What would be the extent of difference on residues on the planes' interiors and exteriors?
- What is the nature of TCDD's physicochemical properties? How would they influence human exposures from herbicide residues on the aircrafts' interiors? How would they influence the content of samples obtained over an extended period of time? Should these physicochemical properties be considered when interpreting the sampling results?
- What environmental factors or activities in the C-123 could have affected the stability of TCDD in the interior of a plane?
- How might TCDD in the surface residues be transferred to dust? What conditions might promote or decrease that process?
- What solvents were used in gathering surface wipes in each period of sampling? Are there any implications for the comparability of the samples?
- What do you think would constitute representative sample(s) for estimating the TCDD exposure of the C-123 Reservists, and why? What combination of available sampling data comes closest to this standard?
- Do you have any opinions or thoughts as to why the 1994 and 1995 samples from "Patches" are so different?

- Under what conditions were the air samples collected (plane on ground with or without door open; plane in flight)?

Modeling with Existing Data

- What is the plausible range of values that could be used as inputs for each of the parameters in the various models?
- The specific values quoted for Model 1 in Lurker's abstract of 0.92 and 5.4 pg/kg-birthweight (BW)-day for the flight crew and maintainers differ from the results the committee obtained (3.0 for 60 kg and 2.5 for 70 kg BW) from equation 2 and using 42 days/year from Table 4 and 250 days/year. Please go through the calculations for the Model 1 results given in the paper given that we were unable to reproduce it from the input parameters given in Table 4 using equation 2.
- When modeling ingestion, what would you consider the most appropriate estimate and the plausible range for:
  - hand to mouth frequency and
  - transfer of TCDD from hand to mouth (for eating food, such as a sandwich, on a flight)?
- How do the assumptions governing TCDD ingestion applied in Lurker et al. (2014) compare with those used in the National Research Council (1988) approach to establishing reentry criteria after polychlorinated biphenyl (PCB) transformer fires? What is the impact on resulting estimates?
- Please explain how the physicochemical properties of TCDD would, or would not, make the application of Model 3 by Lurker et al. (2014) appropriate.

Interpretations of Resulting Exposure Estimates

- What are your opinions of the applicability of various existing health guidelines for TCDD for the case of the AF Reservists who served on C-123s that had previously been used to spray herbicides in Vietnam?
- What existing guidelines would be most appropriate for application to this situation?

Appendix B

History and Sampling of C-123s in the United States After Spraying Herbicides in Vietnam

(Shaded entries are C-123s that were sampled for TCDD)

TABLE B-1 Operation Ranch Hand C-123s Identified in Historical Records[a]

UC-123 Tail #[b]	Squadron Assignment, Museum/Year (if known)	Fate of C-123
54-558	4500th ABW, MAP	Sold to Royal Thai Air Force (Thailand), 1971
54-570	4500th ABW, MAP	Sold to Royal Thai Air Force (Thailand), 1971
54-575	4500th ABW, MAP	Sold to Royal Thai Air Force (Thailand), 1971
54-576	12th SOS (Vietnam, no date); 56th SOW (Thailand, no date); 405th Fighter Wing (The Philippines, no date); South Vietnamese Air Force (1971); MASDC (no date); AFLC (1972); MAP	Sold to Royal Thai Air Force (Thailand), 1973
54-577	12th SOS (Vietnam, no date); 315th TAW (Vietnam, no date); Vietnam Air Force (no date); MASDC (no date); AFLC (no date); Air America (1973); MAP	Sold to Royal Lao Air Force, 1973
54-578	12th SOS (Vietnam, no date); 56th SOW (Thailand, no date); MAP	Sold to South Vietnamese Air Force, 1973
54-584	12th SOS (Vietnam, no date); 315th TAW (Vietnam, no date); Vietnam Air Force (1971); MASDC (no date); AFLC (no date); MAP	Sold to Royal Thai Air Force (Thailand), 1973
54-586	12th SOS (Vietnam, 1968–1970); 315th TAW (Vietnam, no date); MASDC (1970); AFLC (no date); 911 TAG (PA, 1972); 731st TAS (MA, 1981); retired from service 1982	**Destroyed at Davis-Monthan AFB, AZ, 2010**

continued

TABLE B-1 Continued

UC-123 Tail #[b]	Squadron Assignment, Museum/Year (if known)	Fate of C-123
54-588	12th ACS	Crashed/lost, Vietnam, 1962
54-589	12th SOS (Vietnam, no date); 315th TAW (Vietnam, no date); MASDC (no date); MAP	Sold to Royal Thai Air Force (Thailand), no date; records show it was later destroyed in combat
54-591	12th SOS (Vietnam, no date); 315th TAW (Vietnam, no date); Vietnam Air Force (no date); MASDC (no date); MAP	Sold to Philippines Air Force, 1970
54-597	12th ACS	Crashed/lost, Vietnam, 1966
54-602	1st SOS	Crashed/lost, Florida, 1968
54-605	12th SOS (Vietnam, 1966–1968), 315th TAW (Vietnam, no date); MASDC (1970); AFLC (1971); 907th TAG (OH, 1972); 355th TAS (no year); 356th (OH, 1973); retired from service 1984	**Destroyed at Davis-Monthan AFB, AZ, 2010**
54-607	12th SOS (Vietnam, 1966–1969); 315th TAW (Vietnam, no date); MASDC (1971); AFLC (1971); 1st SOW (FL, no year); 24th SOW (Panama, 1973); 907th TAG (OH, 1975); 355th TAS (OH, no year); 356th (OH, no year); 439th AW and 731st TAS (MA, 1976); retired from service 1982	**Destroyed at Davis-Monthan AFB, AZ, 2010**
54-611	12th ACS	Crashed/lost, Loas, 1967
54-618	12th SOS (Vietnam, 1966–1969); 309th SOS (Vietnam, no year); 315th TAW (Vietnam, no year); MASDC (1970); AFLC (1971); ADTC (FL, no year); 302nd TAW, 906th TAG, and 355th TAS (1972–1981, OH); retired from service 1982	**Destroyed at Davis-Monthan AFB, AZ, 2010**
54-621	19th ACS	Crashed/lost, Vietnam, 1967
54-628	12th SOS (Vietnam, 1966–1968); 309th SOS (Vietnam, 1969); 315th TAW (Vietnam, no year); MASDC (1970); AFLC (1971); 355th TAS (OH, no date); retired from service 1982	**Destroyed at Davis-Monthan AFB, AZ, 2010**
54-630	12th ACS	Crashed/lost, Vietnam, 1967
54-633	12th SOS (Vietnam, no date); 315th TAW (Vietnam, no date); MASDC (no date); AFLC (no date); 1st SOW (FL, no date); 906th TAG, 907th TAG, and 355th TAS (OH, no dates); retired from service 1982	*Retired for preservation—Museum of Aviation, Robins AFB, GA, 1984*
54-658	12th SOS (Vietnam, no date); 315th TAW (Vietnam, no date); MASDC (1970); AFLC (no date); 24th SOW (Panama, no date); 906th TAG and 355th TAS (OH, no dates); retired from service 1982	*Retired for preservation—Mobility Command Museum, Dover AFB, DE, 1987*

TABLE B-1 Continued

UC-123 Tail #[b]	Squadron Assignment, Museum/Year (if known)	Fate of C-123
54-693	12th SOS (Vietnam, 1967–1968); 309th SOS (Vietnam, 1969); 315th TAW (Vietnam); MASDC (1970); AFLC (1971); 1st SOW (FL, no date); 355th TAS and 356th TAS (OH, no date); retired from service 1982	**Destroyed at Davis-Monthan AFB, AZ, 2010**
54-701	12th SOS (Vietnam, 1968–1970), 309th SOS (Taiwan, 1969); 315th TAW (Vietnam, no date); MASDC (1970); AFLC (1970); 4500th ABW (VA, 1970); 906th TAG, 355th TAS and 356th TAS (OH, no dates); retired from service 1982	**Destroyed at Davis-Monthan AFB, AZ, 2010**
55-4511	12th SOS (Vietnam, 1968); 315th TAW (Vietnam, no date); MASDC (no date); AFLC (no date); MAP	Republic of Korea, no year
55-4520	12th SOS (Vietnam, 1968–1969); 310th SOS (Taiwan, 1969); 315th TAW (Vietnam, no date); MASDC (1970); AFLC (1971); 51st ABW (South Korea, no date); 56th ABW (AZ, no date); 907th TAG (OH, no date); 356th TAS (OH, no date); retired from service 1981	**Destroyed at Davis-Monthan AFB, AZ, 2010**
55-4532	12th SOS (Vietnam, 1968–1970); 310th SOS (Taiwan, no date); 315th TAW (Vietnam, 1970); MASDC (1970); 24th SOW (Panama, 1970); AMARC (1970); AFLC (1971); 911th TAG (PA, no date); retired from service 1980	**Destroyed at Davis-Monthan AFB, AZ, 2010**
55-4547	12th SOS (Vietnam, 1968–1969); 310th TAW (Taiwan, 1969); 315th TAW (Vietnam, no date); MASDC (1970); AFLC (no date); 4500th ABW (VA, 1970); 906th TAG, 355th TAS, and 356th TAS (OH, no date); retired from service 1986	**Destroyed at Davis-Monthan AFB, AZ, 2010**
55-4570	12th SOS and 311th SOS (Vietnam, 1968–1969); 315th TAW (Vietnam, no date); MASDC (1970); AFLC (no date); 51st ABW (Korea, no date); 907th TAG (OH, no date); retired to AMARC (no date); MAP	Royal Thai Air Force (Thailand), 1975 *(currently located in Chiang Mai Museum, Thailand)*
55-4571	12th SOS (Vietnam, 1968–1969); 310th TAW (Taiwan, 1969); 315th TAW (Vietnam, no date); MASDC (1970); AFLC (no date); 24th SOW (Panama, no date); 907th TAG, 355th TAS, and 356th TAS (OH, no date); retired from service 1986	**Destroyed at Davis-Monthan AFB, AZ, 2010**
55-4577	12th SOS (Vietnam, 1967–1968); 310th SOS (Taiwan, no date); 315th TAW (Vietnam, no date); 911th TAG and 758th TAS (PA, 1972); MASDC (1980)	**Destroyed at Davis-Monthan AFB, AZ, 2010**

continued

TABLE B-1 Continued

UC-123 Tail #[b]	Squadron Assignment, Museum/Year (if known)	Fate of C-123
56-4362 ("Patches")	346th TCS (NC, 1961); ORH (Vietnam, 1962); 4500th ABW (VA, 1962); 315th Air Division Headquarters, 2nd Division (Vietnam, 1963); 377th CSG (Vietnam, 1966); 315th ACW (Vietnam, 1966 [converted to UC-123 in MD, 1968]); 315th TAW (Vietnam, 1968 [converted to insecticide sprayer—Operation Flyswatter]); 377th (Vietnam, 1972); MASDC (1972); 911th TAG (PA, no date); 901st TAG and 731st TAS (MA, 1972)	*Retired for preservation—US Air Force Museum, Wright-Patterson, AFB, OH, 1980*
56-4368	464th TCW	Crashed/lost, Vietnam, 1962
56-4370	464th TCW	Crashed/lost, Vietnam, 1962
56-4371	12th SOS (Vietnam, no date); 315th TAW (Vietnam, no date); MASDC (1970); AFLC (1971); 906th TAG (OH, no date); 355th TAS (OH, 1975); retired from service 1982	**Destroyed at Davis-Monthan AFB, AZ, 2010**
56-4373	310th TAS	Crashed/lost, Vietnam, 1971
56-4378	309th ACS	Crashed/lost, Vietnam, 1966
56-4384	12th SOS (Vietnam, no date); 310th SOS (1969); 315th TAW (Vietnam, no date); MASDC (no date); AFLC (no date); MASDC (no date); MAP	Year and country undisclosed
57-6289	12th SOS (Vietnam, no date); 315th TAW (Vietnam, no date); 405 Fighter Wing (The Philippines, no date); MASDC (1970); Vietnam Air Force (1971); AFLC (1973); MASDC (no date); MAP	Royal Thai Air Force (Thailand), 1973
57-6291	12th SOS (Vietnam, no date); 315th SOW (Vietnam, no date); MASDC (1970); AFLC (no date); 302nd TAW, 906th TAG, and 355th TAS (OH, no dates)	Crashed, Oklahoma, 1980

[a] C-123 aircraft tail #'s 54-583, 54-585, 54-635, 54-685, and 55-4544 were *excluded* from this table. Each of these aircraft were identified as Operation Ranch Hand planes in some recent historical documents provided by the VA (Young and Young, 2013, 2014a,b); however, although these C-123 aircraft were stationed with the 12th SOS in Vietnam (Operation Ranch Hand), the flight records for these aircraft do not indicate that they were used for herbicide missions (USAF, 2009a). Tail #56-4375, nicknamed "The White Whale" was used for VIP transport, not herbicide missions, and was also excluded from this table.

[b] C-123 aircraft tail numbers that are in bold were destroyed and recycled in 2010.

SOURCES: Information compiled from Alvin L. Young, A.L. Young Consulting, Inc., personal communication, May 5, 2014; Carter, 2013; Young, 2014; Young and Young, 2014a,b.

ABBREVIATIONS: ABW, Air Base Wing; ACG, Air Commando Group; ACS, Air Commando Squadron; ACW, Air Command Wing; ADTC, Armament Development and Test Center (Eglin Air Force Base, FL); AFB, Air Force base; AFLC, Air Force Logistic Command (Hayes Aircraft Facility, Napier Field, Dothan, AL); AMARC, Aerospace Maintenance and Regeneration Center (Davis-Monthan Air Force Base, Tucson, AZ); CSG, Combat Support Group; MASDC, Military Aircraft Storage and Disposal Center (Davis-Monthan Air Force Base, Tucson, AZ); SOS, Special Operations Squadron; SOW, Special Operations Wing; TAG, Tactical Air Group; TAS, Tactical Airlift Squadron; TAW, Tactical Air Wing; TCS, Troop Carrier Squadron; TCW, Troop Carrier Wing.

TABLE B-2 Sampling of C-123s in the United States After Spraying Herbicides in Vietnam

Date	Event	Plane	Sampling	Other
03/09/1979 (Report dated 09/1979)	Sampling—Westover AFB (to determine the source of bad odors)	"Patches"	**3 Air Samples**—(2,4-D and 2,4,5-T = 0.243 mg/m^3 to 0.428 mg/m^3); TLV = 10 mg/m^3 **1 Paint Scraping from cargo tie-down rings (& 1 residue sample lost)** (detection limit 60 µg/kg) 2,4-D = < 60 µg/kg; 2,4,5-T = < 60 µg/kg • 2,4-D Butyl Ester µg/kg (AO) = < 60 • 2,4-D Isooctyl Ester µg/kg (AOII) ≈ 92 • 2,4,5-T Butyl Ester µg/kg (AO) ≈149 • 2,4,5-T Isooctyl Ester µg/kg (AOII) = < 60 Malathion µg/kg ≈ 145	Malathion ≈ 145 µg/kg Black residue found in wing was malathion
1994 (date samples taken unclear, request for samples in September; first discussed November 1994)	Wright-Patterson AFB Museum Annex	"Patches"	**Swipes:** 2,3,7,8-TCDD (nanograms/sample): [interior 200 ng/m^2, 1400 ng/m^2] Interior (midship), 14.22098 (TEQ, 14.458) Interior (tail), 2.06846 (TEQ, 2.152) Interior (tail), 2.40728 (TEQ, 2.491) Exterior (wing), 0.04015 (TEQ, 0.041 [4.1 ng/m^2]) Exterior (wing), 0.00255 (TEQ, 0.003 [0.3 ng/m^2]) Also values for PCDD, PCDF, etc.	Document describes plane as "highly contaminated" (Samples analyzed by Pace Incorporated Environmental Laboratories)

continued

TABLE B-2 Continued

Date	Event	Plane	Sampling	Other
09/13/1995	Sampling—Wright-Patterson AFB Museum Annex (sampling done by OHM Remediation Services, Corp.)	"Patches"	**49 surface wipes (TCDD)** Composite A2: 0 ng/600 cm^2 *Interior Front Port* Composite A3: 3.2 ng/400 cm^2 [53 ng/m^2] (figures as noted in Appendix B, corrected from 3.2 ng/600 cm^2) *Inside inspection ports on rear bottom of aircraft (exterior) (described in 11/17 memo as rear of cargo bay); report says "inspection ports which tested positive are below the same area of the interior which was hot"* Composite A5: 0 ng/600 cm^2 *Interior Front Starboard* Composite A6: 0 ng/600 cm^2 *Interior Center Port* Composite A7: 0 ng/600 cm^2 *Interior Center Starboard* Composite A8 1.8 ng/600 cm^2 [45 ng/m^2] (figures as noted in Appendix B, corrected from 1.8 ng/400 cm^2) *Interior Rear* (rear interior of cargo bay) No dioxin found on exterior of plane or spray equipment	WESTON Laboratories (ng/m^2 measurements from UC = 123K Sampling and Analysis Plan, February 2009)
11/17/1995	Wright-Patterson AFB Museum Annex (proposal for decontamination)	"Patches"	A *proposal* OHM Remediation Services, Corp.—once aircraft wiped down 3 times, "175 wipe samples will be taken plus 10 percent for quality control"	

07/1996	Wright-Patterson AFB Museum Annex (proposal for decontamination)	“Patches”	New *proposal* from OHM Remediation Services, Corp.—16 wipe samples will be taken including those for quality control, proposes to composite the wipes from designated sections of the grid before analysis is performed by USEPA Method 8280; four composite samples will be analyzed, representing a 2,500 cm^2 area
09/1996	Sampling 309th Aerospace Maintenance and Regeneration Group (AMARG—formerly AMARC), Davis-Monthan AFB, AZ	17 planes (5 without documentation of service in Operation Ranch Hand)	17 planes swipe sampled for 2,4-D and 2,4,5-T prior to sale; 2 samples per plane (from inboard spray fittings and floor underneath fittings). Swipes collected on moist Whatman glass filters from 6 × 6 areas “of the floor located under the spray line caps” and “inside the spray line” *14 of 17 samples had detectable herbicides* *(2.2 μg/swipe to 960 μg/swipe)*
02/1997	Wright-Patterson AFB Museum Annex	“Patches”	Memo stating that “Patches” is now washed and de-contaminated and open for employee and public access (aircraft sampled by OHM Remediation Services, Corp. after cleaning . . . no dioxin contamination detected [cleanup action level of 25 ng/m^2])

continued

Date	Event	Plane	Sampling	Other
02/18–19/2009 (USAF, 2009b)	AMARG	4 Planes Tail #'s *54-585* (no detect in 1996) (herbicide sprayer but not RH according to AMARG and Dr. Paul Cecil); *55-4571* (> 25 µg/wipe, 1996) (RH according to AMARG); *55-4532* (> 25 µg/wipe 1996) (RH according to AMARG); *55-4544* (no detect in 1996) (herbicide sprayer but not RH according to AMARG and Dr. Paul Cecil)	**<u>124 wipe samples</u>** (not including 2 lost samples); 100 square cm area, hexane used for dioxin/furan samples and water for herbicide samples *Wipe Sampling Results:* No detectable AO constituents on exterior • 2,4-D and 2,4,5-T—very low, no significant risk (1,600 and 1100 µg/m^2, respectively) (level of concern, 100,000 µg/m) • 2,4-D (*55-4571*): 587 µg/m^2; 95% UCL = 911 µg/m^2 in interior • 2,4-D (55-4532): 453 µg/m^2; 95% UCL = 781 µg/m^2 in interior • 2,4,5-T (*55-4571*): 518 µg/m^2; 95% UCL = 698 µg/m^2 in interior • 2,4, 5-T (55-4532): 502 µg/m^2; 95% UCL = 815 µg/m^2 in interior 2 aircraft (*55-4544*, *54-0585*) had trace levels of dioxin/furans on interior floor locations (max 3.9 ng/m^2 TEQ [risk-based screening level value, 23 ng/m^2]) and non-detect levels or all other surfaces 2 aircraft had low level dioxin/furans on all interior surfaces (*55-4571*—14.95 ng/m^2 TEQ; *5504532*—18.2 ng/m^2 TEQ with 95% UCLs of 21.7 and 24.7 ng/m^2); considered to have low-level contamination that does not pose a risk for personnel for recycling activities. Levels inside spray tank were very high **<u>16 air samples</u>**: 2,4-D and 2,4,5-T collected in fuselage with pump and glass fiber filter at a rate of 2L/minute for 60 minutes. Dioxins/furans collected on a foam plug at 4L/minute for ~ 4 hours (testing for conditions for unprotected workers cleaning out debris from planes … not flying in planes. *Air Sampling Results:* No detectable AO constituents in any air samples	Samples conducted to obtain data "to assess what controls (if any, may be needed to ensure protection of the health and safety of recycling personnel" Samples set to TestAmerica analytical laboratories

NOTES: 2,4-D, 2,4-dichlorophenoxy acetic acid; 2,4,5-T, 2,4,5-trichlorophenoxyacetic acid; AFB, Air Force Base; AMARC, Aircraft Maintenance and Regeneration Center; AMARG, Aerospace Maintenance and Regeneration Group; AO, Agent Orange (50% *n*-butyl ester of 2,4-D, 50% *n*-butyl ester of 2,4,5-T); AOII, Agent Orange II (50% *n*-butyl ester of 2,4-D, 50% *n*-isooctyl ester of 2,4,5-T); MASDC, Military Aircraft Storage and Disposal Center; nd, not detected; PCDD, polychlorinated dibenzo-*p*-dioxin; PCDF, polychlorinated dibenzofuran; RH, Ranch Hand; TCDD, 2,3,7,8-trichlorodibenzo-*p*-dioxin; TEQ, Toxicity Equivalency Quotient; USAF, United States Air Force; USEPA, United States Environmental Protection Agency.
AMARG refers to the 309th Aerospace Maintenance and Regeneration Group, often called *The Boneyard*, is a US Air Force aircraft and missile storage and maintenance facility in Tucson, Arizona, located on Davis-Monthan Air Force Base.
AMARG was previously Aerospace Maintenance and Regeneration Center, AMARC, the Military Aircraft Storage and Disposal Center, MASDC, and started life after World War II as the 3040th Aircraft Storage Group.

Appendix C

Committee Biographies

Robert F. Herrick, Sc.D. (*Chair*), is a senior lecturer on occupational hygiene at the Harvard School of Public Health. His educational background includes a B.A. degree in chemistry from the College of Wooster, an M.S. in Environmental Health Science from the University of Michigan, and a Doctor of Science in Industrial Hygiene from the Harvard School of Public Health. He is certified in the comprehensive practice of industrial hygiene. His research interests are centered on the assessment of exposure as a cause of occupational and environmental disease. He has conducted research on the development of methods to measure the biologically active characteristics of reactive aerosols, and on studies of work processes in the construction and semiconductor industries to develop task-based models to identify and control the primary sources of worker exposures. He has also investigated exposures and biomarkers of polychlorinated biphenyl (PCB) exposures to workers in PCB-contaminated buildings. Dr. Herrick is Past Chair of the American Conference of Governmental Industrial Hygienists (ACGIH), and Past President of the International Occupational Hygiene Association. Prior to joining the faculty at the Harvard School of Public Health, Dr. Herrick spent 17 years at the National Institute for Occupational Safety and Health (NIOSH) where he conducted occupational health research. Dr. Herrick also previously served on the Institute of Medicine Committee to Review the Health Effects of Vietnam Veterans of Exposure to Herbicides—Second and Third Biennial Updates as well as the Committee for a Review of Evidence Regarding Link between Exposure to Agent Orange and Diabetes.

Robert Canales, Ph.D., M.S., is an assistant professor in the Community, Environment and Policy Division at the Mel & Enid Zuckerman School of Public

Health at the University of Arizona. He received his M.S. in statistics and his Ph.D. in environmental engineering and science from Stanford University and was a post-doctoral fellow at the Harvard School of Public Health. Dr. Canales applies principles in the natural sciences and mathematics to explore environmental health issues, particularly human exposure to environmental contaminants. With a background in environmental engineering, public health, and statistics, his research focuses on creating models/simulations and exploring data to improve human health, and has included a variety of projects: modeling the fate and transport of contaminants in indoor environments, simulating children's behavior and contaminant intake levels, and distinguishing demographic variables for identifying households with high indoor pesticide concentrations, to name a few.

Kenny S. Crump, Ph.D., is currently serving as an independent consultant, having retired as a principal with Environ Corporation in 2007. He has more than 35 years of experience in assessing risk related to exposure to toxic materials. He has served on science advisory boards of the Environmental Protection Agency, the National Center for Toxicological Research, the Mickey Leland National Urban Air Toxics Research Center, and the National Institute of Environmental Health Sciences. His research interests are in the areas of biostatistics, health risk assessment, and analysis of epidemiological data. Statistical models for assessing risk developed by Dr. Crump have been widely used by regulatory agencies and private groups. These include the Linearized Multistage Model and the benchmark methodology. Dr. Crump has participated in risk assessments of many substances, including asbestos, benzene, manganese, and mercury. He received his Ph.D. in Mathematics from Montana State University, his M.A. in Mathematics from the University of Denver, and his B.S. in Electrical Engineering from Louisiana Tech University. He was previously a member of the National Academies Standing Committee on Risk Analysis Issues and Reviews, the Committee on Risk Assessment Methodology, and the Committee on Institutional Means for Assessment of Risks to Public Health.

Melissa Gonzales, Ph.D., is an associate professor in the Division of Epidemiology and the University of New Mexico (UNM). She received her Ph.D. in environmental health at the University of California, Berkeley, School of Public Health, and prior to that she earned a masters degree in toxicology/industrial hygiene at the University of Arizona, College of Pharmacy. She joined the Division of Epidemiology, Biostatistics, and Preventive Medicine at the UNM School of Medicine in 2002. She was recruited from the US Environmental Protection Agency (EPA), where she had been a postdoctoral research fellow in the Epidemiology and Biomarkers Branch of the National Health and Environmental Effects Research Laboratory, EPA Office of Research and Development. While at EPA, she was the co-investigator of the El Paso Children's Health Study, and senior staff to the US chair of the US–Mexico Border 21 Environmental Health

Workgroup. Dr. Gonzales' research focuses on understanding the contribution of environmental exposures to chronic illnesses such as asthma and cancer. Her work includes the Albuquerque Hispanic Moms Study, the Zuni Exposure Study, the Colorectal Disease Prevention Study and the University of New Mexico–University of Texas El Paso study of asthma and respiratory health among children living on the US–Mexico border (ARCH). Dr. Gonzales is currently the assistant program director for the UNM Preventive Medicine Residency Program, director of the environmental health core in the UNM Health Disparities Research Center, and a founding member of the UNM Metal Exposure Toxicity Assessment on Tribal Lands in the Southwest (METALS) Research Program, where she leads initiatives to reduce exposure uncertainty in risk assessment and prioritization strategies for complex environmental exposures.

John C. Kissel, Ph.D., PE, is professor of Environmental and Occupational Health Sciences at the University of Washington. Dr. Kissel is an environmental engineer whose research focuses on human exposure to environmental contaminants. He is a former President and Councilor of the International Society of Exposure Science and former chair of the Exposure Assessment Specialty Group of the Society for Risk Analysis. He is also an ad hoc member of the US Environmental Protection Agency (EPA) Federal Insecticide, Fungicide and Rodenticide Act Science Advisory Panel and served as a member of a National Academy of Sciences/National Research Council committee examining Superfund cleanup of mining wastes in the Coeur d'Alene River Basin of northern Idaho. Dr. Kissel has conducted research funded by EPA, the National Institute of Occupational Safety and Health, the US Department of Energy, and the US Department of Defense via the Strategic Environmental Research and Development Program.

Linda A. McCauley, Ph.D., R.N., F.A.A.N., F.A.A.O.H.N., is dean and professor at Emory University's Nell Hodgson Woodruff School of Nursing, and Professor in the Department of Environmental Health at the Rollins School of Public Health. Dr. McCauley is a nationally recognized leader in nursing education and is a national leader in research on environmental exposures and health hazards among vulnerable populations, including workers and young children. Dr. McCauley has been awarded research funding from the National Institutes of Health, the Centers for Disease Control and Prevention, the US Department of Defense, and the US Department of Veterans Affairs. Her research has resulted in numerous publications, ongoing consultations, leadership on occupational and environmental advisory panels, and testimony to governmental oversight bodies. Dr. McCauley is a fellow of the American Academy of Occupational Health Nurses and the American Academy of Nursing. She is a member of the American College of Occupational and Environmental Medicine, the Sigma Theta Tau Honorary Nursing Society, the American Nurses Association, the American Public Health Association, and the Institute of Medicine. She currently serves on the executive committee as one of the founding leaders for the Future of Nursing: Campaign for Action initiative in Georgia. Dr. McCauley received her bachelor's degree in nursing from the University of North Carolina at Chapel Hill, her master's degree in nursing from Emory University, and her Ph.D. in environmental health from the University of Cincinnati.

Clifford P. Weisel, Ph.D., is a professor in the Exposure Science Division of the Department of Environmental and Occupational Medicine of the Robert Wood Johnson Medical School/Rutgers University, where he has been of the faculty since 1989. He also holds appointments on the graduate faculty of Environmental Sciences and School of Public Health at Rutgers University. He is the Deputy Director of the Exposure Science Division of the Environmental and Occupational Health Sciences Institute and Director of the Doctoral Degree Program in Exposure Sciences. Dr. Weisel research areas include understanding exposure to chemical agents in various modes of transportation including aircraft, multi-route exposures to environmental contaminants and their associated adverse health effects, and the development and application of biomarkers of exposure. He is currently a scientific member of the Federal Aviation Administration Center of Excellence on Airliner Cabin Environment Research. He has examined the relationship among indoor, outdoor and personal exposure to air pollutants; documented the importance of inhalation and dermal exposure to contaminants, and examined exposure and health issues related to disinfection by products, in water. He is the past president of the International Society of Exposure Science and has served on numerous international and national advisory committees, workshops and advisory review panels for the US Environmental Protection Agency, National Institute of Environmental Health Sciences, Centers for Disease Control and Prevention, state governmental agencies, environmental groups, and private industry. He has been an associate editor of the *Journal of Exposure Science and Environmental Epidemiology*. He was awarded the Jerome J. Wesolowski Award in 2013 by the International Society of Exposure Science in recognition of outstanding contributions to the knowledge and practice of human exposure science. Dr. Weisel has authored or co-authored more than 100 peer-reviewed publications and book chapters and co-authored with Paul Lioy the book *Exposure Science: Basic Principles and Applications* published in 2014. He previously served on the Institute of Medicine Committee to Review the Health Effects in Vietnam Veterans of Exposure to Herbicides.